THE

mom's

GUIDE TO

growing your
family green

THE

mom's

GUIDE TO

growing your
family green

SAVING THE EARTH BEGINS AT HOME

TERRA WELLINGTON

A Stonesong Press Book

St. Martin's Griffin
New York

I dedicate this book to my children—
may you have a beautiful future.

And to my husband—
thank you for always
believing in me.

THE MOM'S GUIDE TO GROWING YOUR FAMILY GREEN. Copyright © 2009 by Terra Wellington and The Stonesong Press, LLC. All rights reserved. Printed in the United States of America. For information, address St. Martin's Press, 175 Fifth Avenue, New York, N.Y. 10010.

NFRC label on page 15 courtesy of the NFRC; UL logo on page 39 courtesy of Underwriters Laboratories Inc.; WaterSense logo on page 49, Energy Star logo on page 64, U.S. EPA logo on page 100, and GreenScapes logo on page 128 courtesy of U.S. Environmental Protection Agency; EnergyGuide label on page 66 courtesy of Federal Trade Commission; KCMA logo on page 70 courtesy of Kitchen Cabinet Manufacturers Association; recycling logos on pages 85–86 courtesy of Packing Graphics Co.; Green Seal logo on page 100 courtesy of Green Seal; EcoLogo on page 100 courtesy of TerraChoice Environmental Marketing, Inc.; Certified Humane logo on page 161 courtesy of Humane Farm Animal Care; Food Alliance Certified logo on page 161 courtesy of Food Alliance; Leaping Bunny logo on page 168 courtesy of the Coalition for Consumer Information on Cosmetics; USDA Organic logo on page 171 courtesy of U.S. Department of Agriculture; Veriflora logo on page 172 courtesy of Scientific Certification Systems; Marine Stewardship Council logo on page 177 courtesy of Marine Stewardship Council; FSC logo on page 228 courtesy of the Forest Stewardship Council.

A Stonesong Press Book

www.stmartins.com

Book design by Stephanie Huntwork

ISBN-13: 978-0-312-38473-9
ISBN-10: 0-312-38473-4

First Edition: March 2009

10 9 8 7 6 5 4 3 2 1

Interior text printed on SFI-certified paper, 20% recycled content.

CONTENTS

ACKNOWLEDGMENTS

Writing this book has been a journey for me. In the process of compiling this manuscript, I have been fortunate to be privy to information and interviews that have changed my life. I'm just one person trying to make a difference, just like all of you. And one of the most striking feelings I have had about penning this guidebook is how much I love and appreciate all that the earth has given me. I have seen many marvelous things in my life—memorable national parks, breathtaking coastlines and beaches, fascinating animals, the miracle of the growth of a seed into a plant, and long summer days in my green backyard as a child.

One of my earliest childhood memories is the fun I had flipping up my feet against an old-growth tree in the backyard and watching the white puffballed clouds traipse through the sky; I did what any child without video games and computers would do—turn those clouds into images and make up stories. I want to leave that same multicolored, sweet legacy for my children. I want them to have a clean and beautiful world to embrace for themselves, their children, and their children's children after that. I feel strongly about this not only for tangible survival reasons but also because of spiritual and emotional reasons. Ask yourself if you do not feel the same way. I bet you do.

I want to give special thanks to Alison Fargis at the Stonesong Press, who believed in me from the beginning. If every author were so privileged! She and her brilliant team, including Katie Feiereisel, have championed my ideas and have made this book possible. I am grateful to Sheila Curry Oakes and Alyse Diamond at St. Martin's Press for caring enough about the environment and families to publish this book. I appreciate the contributions of the Alliance to Save Energy, lighting expert Andris Kasparovics, the National Wildlife Federation, Peter Sinsheimer at Occidental College, Martin Wolf of Seventh Generation, Shelley Flint at the U.S. Humane Society, Patricia Calkins with Xerox, Kreigh Hampel with the Burbank Recycling Center, Ron Mader at Planeta.com, and Disney-Family.com. Both Algalita's president John Fentis and Environmental Defense Fund's John Balbus were kind enough to explain many important issues to me. And I wish to thank Deron Lovaas at the Natural Resources Defense Council for his assistance in helping me define the fuel section—an emerging and evolving issue that confronts us all—as well as Alexandra Kennaugh's time in talking with me about issues that all families face regarding the environment and consumer products. Many other companies have contributed information and resources for this book, and I appreciate all their time and effort. I also appreciate the assistance of Don MacDonald and Marc Berkman from my congressional representative Brad Sherman's office in Washington, D.C. They served as a vital liaison between me and the U.S. Environmental Protection Agency.

Finally, and most important, I am grateful for the support of my family. My kids are patient when I ask them to take out the recycling, come to the farmers' market with me, or spend some time outside—they go purely on faith that a break from video gaming can bring them something beneficial. And my always-supportive husband has championed all my eco initiatives: I even got him to stir the compost pile!

growing your family green
begins with *you*

I've been a television contributor on healthy living and consumer wellness topics for many years. But even with all that I know about creating and maintaining a healthy lifestyle, nothing has such broad quality-of-life implications as how we take care of the environment. Our environment provides us the air we breathe, the food we eat, the products we buy, the recreation and beauty we enjoy, the clean water we need, and a carefully constructed set of ecosystems that keep everything in check.

The protection of this environment—and how your health, safety, and happiness relate to that protection—is why I have written this book. I want to raise your level of awareness and change your thinking, because this is literally how you will save your life and your children's lives. That is how important this book is.

The environment is *not* something "out there"; rather, you and the environment coexist and what happens to the environment also happens to you. You and your family now live in a world that *demands that you pay attention to it* instead of just existing in it. No matter what are your current beliefs about climate change or greenhouse gases, the indisputable facts are that the earth is warming, being polluted, and losing a great deal of what was once pristine. Because of this, it is important that all of us find a way to contribute to reversing these negative trends—for ourselves and our children. If we don't, then in a relatively short period of time (just a few decades) you won't have clean air and water, much of your food options will disappear, there will be escalating illness and safety issues due to pollution, weather-related disasters will wreck havoc on your life, whole ecosystems on land and in water will collapse, and many of the recreational places you love and enjoy will either take a dramatic change for the worse or no longer exist at all. Inherent in all of this are also economic problems—loss of jobs, loss of property, increased health-care costs, and much higher prices for food, water, and energy.

Yes, the thought of all this happening in the next few decades *is* scary, and it is easy to think that one person cannot make a difference. But change has to start somewhere, and the best place begins with the family. Families are the threads that knit us together and provide little microworlds of change and influence that ripple through humanity across the globe. We love our families. We want to keep them safe. This is why change needs to begin with moms. With us at the helm, we can each make a difference. Through the information you will learn in this book, you can help keep your family from harm and save the environment from further damage. You are where greening starts.

TODAY'S HEALTH AND TOMORROW'S FUTURE, INTER-TWINED >> In a survey of more than 8,000 moms and dads, DisneyFamily.com learned these results:

- More than 80 percent of respondents said the environment was important to them.
- The most important issues were clean water, recycling and reducing waste, and air pollution.
- The top two reasons parents were concerned about the environment was that they were looking out for the future of their children (80 percent) and because the health of their family was important to them (75 percent).
- And 55 percent said their child was very aware of environmental issues.

live with both eyes open

John Balbus is the chief health scientist for the Environmental Defense Fund (www.edf.org), one of the most important environmental groups in the world. He says that when it comes to the environment, you need to determine who you want to listen to: "Religious leaders are increasingly speaking with one voice and have deep concern about the [environmental] path that we're on. Clearly, you should pay attention to the voice of the scientific consensus. But you should also be listening to the voice of your children." Many children are scared and angry that our planet is in the torn-down shape it's in, and they want their parents to find a solution.

When it comes to solutions, Balbus says: "I like the concept of living with both eyes open. It is the idea of trying to educate yourself [about] where things come from, what it takes to make them, what kinds of resources are needed to get them there—and then it's really a question of being comfortable and confident that the small incremental changes that you might make are going to make a difference."

getting your family on board

Because most parents have limited time and budgets, an understandable reaction is, "I have too much on my plate already. How can I possibly add more to my to-do list?" Have no fear. All the how-to's in this book are about raising your family green in a *practical way*—so that it becomes part of your lifestyle. Trust me: It is doable.

I can still remember the day our first curbside recycling bin was delivered to my home with a note from the city about what to put in it and when recyclables would be collected. It's hard to believe that initially we couldn't remember what went in the bin and what went in the trash. It seemed like such a chore. Today, however, we separate our recycling from our other trash without a second thought. It has become a part of our lifestyle.

This book is all about creating lifestyle changes. Some of these changes don't add more to your plate, they just change *how* you do things. Other changes ask you to care more, and donate what time and resources you have available. This is how you create meaningful change in your home, your community, and beyond—one person making a difference in a real way.

The easiest way to increase your family's environmental awareness and action is to make lifestyle changes that don't create more work for you, but rather change the way you do the things you already do. This way, you can choose the activities that your time, budget, and interests allow. And if you can make little changes a bit at a time—how you do things, what you buy, and how you influence others—they can add up to big benefits for you, your family, your community, and the world. Not only will this approach reward you and your family with both short- and long-term benefits, but it will also raise the next generation to be healthier and more environmentally conscious adults who will continue to impact their families and communities for the better.

Throughout this book I am going to offer you some easily achievable lifestyle changes and a multitude of ways to become greener. All the tips are written with you—the busy mom—in mind. *You* make the decision on which activities, resources, and information are worth your time and money, and which ones make sense to integrate into your family's life. Maybe you'll choose some options now, then others later. It doesn't have to be done all at once. You can rely on these icons to help you immediately identify benefits, savings, and expenses:

- ✚ health benefits
- ✿ time savings
- ☺ money savings
- ∅ free
- $ minimal expense (less than $50)
- $$ moderate expense ($50–300)
- $$$ expensive ($300–1,000)
- $$$$ investment (more than $1,000)

I will also list products, companies, organizations, and programs that may be of interest to you. While I have tried to seek out the best options available, the reality is that no corporation or their products are perfect. Some companies are environmentally and socially responsible in certain aspects yet perform poorly in other areas of great concern, so choosing which ones to include became a subjective judgment call. Whether they are listed in this book or not, I encourage you to patronize the companies that create less pollution and waste, use more renewable resources, and take their social and ecological responsibility seriously. Far too many consumer-product companies still avoid taking determined steps toward needed change; for the moment, they are willing to ignore that what they produce and how they produce it is destructive and unsustainable. Money is the great determiner of which businesses will survive, so spend it where it counts.

The bottom line is, our earth has limited resources and requires a proactive effort on everyone's part to ensure that it continues to provide for all our needs in a healthy and sustainable way. So let's get started with some simple lifestyle changes that will help you not only care for your family, but also protect the earth.

—Terra Wellington
(www.momsandtheplanet.com)

CHAPTER ONE

earth-friendly energy: taking control of your indoor climate

The majority of your family's life happens in your home. It's where you enjoy holidays, visit with extended family and friends, relax, entertain, eat, and sleep. Because you spend so much time in your home, climate control is an important issue. Moms everywhere should use a green touch when it comes to heating and cooling their homes—heating and cooling account for a large portion of the energy your home uses, and thus a large portion of the money you spend on utilities and of the carbon footprint you leave behind. Take the time to evaluate and improve the methods you use to heat and cool your indoor living areas and you will discover new ways to grow your family green.

a changing world

According to the latest scientific research, if we continue on our destructive path of polluting our environment beyond its capability to renew itself, we can expect climate changes such as periods of extreme drought and precipitation. These climate changes can cause severe economic problems and health risks, changes in the distribution and health of ecosystems, extreme storms that put populations in danger, and more air and water pollution. I, for one, don't want to leave that legacy to my children. *Do you?*

Why do these climate changes happen? In a nutshell, when humans burn coal, oil, and gas (often by way of power plants and transportation, including our cars), create methane gas (through fossil fuel production and raising of livestock), and cut down lots of trees, greenhouse gases are produced. These gases cause global warming when they trap the sun's heat in our atmosphere, which gradually warms our planet's temperature. Because we have produced such a high quantity of these gases over the years, we have caused the earth's overall temperature to rise. This rise in temperature creates climate change. The best known way to reverse this negative impact is to reduce these greenhouse gases (also called emissions) and plant more trees—both of which we can do.

LIFESTYLE ACTION

take stock of your energy

what you need to know

When I pay my bills every month, it's an eye-opening experience to realize just how much power my family uses—and how pricey that energy can be! According to Energy Star, a typical family (mine included) spends approximately $1,900 a year on energy bills, with nearly half of that going to heating and cooling. And if you're like me, you want to reduce this amount. A first step is to find where you might be wasting energy inside your home. Energy Star suggests that better sealing and insulation can save you 10 percent on that bill (that's almost $200 per year). Additionally, you can save another 20 percent by having regular maintenance performed on your cooling system. And programmable thermostats and other energy-saving devices and appliances can help further.

The amount of energy you use is not only directly related to your checkbook, but also to how much you contribute to polluting your environment. We're talking about the air you, I, and our children breathe. In fact, according to the EPA, pollution from homes makes up 17 percent of the greenhouse gases released in this country.

>> The United States is a hungry country when it comes to energy. According to the Population Reference Bureau, we are only 5 percent of the world's population but use over a quarter of nearly every resource produced by the entire planet.

benefits

By reducing your energy usage and paying attention to how you use energy, you can lower your bills and create a healthier environment.

how-to's

Perform a Do-It-Yourself Energy Audit on Your Home ☺

Use my checklist to perform a simple, do-it-yourself energy audit. It will take less than an hour.

> **ENERGY STAR >>** (www.energystar.gov) This is a joint program of the U.S. Environmental Protection Agency and the U.S. Department of Energy to help you save money and protect the environment. The Energy Star label is given to products and services that have met strict energy-saving guidelines.

DO-IT-YOURSELF POWER$MART CHECKLIST
An Action-Based Home-Energy Audit

Energy-Efficient Energy Star Purchases *When your budget allows, look for new or replacement Energy Star-qualified products for energy efficiency.*	Already in Place	House- hold Goal	Date Achieved
1. High-efficiency furnace/air conditioner or heat pump.			
2. Programmable thermostat.			
3. Energy Star-qualified double-pane windows with Low-E coatings and acceptable National Fenestration Rating Council (NFRC) ratings.			
4. Compact and other types of fluorescent light bulbs.			
5. Energy-efficient refrigerator.			
6. Dishwasher that saves water and energy.			

(continued)

DO-IT-YOURSELF POWER$MART CHECKLIST
An Action-Based Home-Energy Audit

	Already in Place	House-hold Goal	Date Achieved
Energy-Efficient Energy Star Purchases *When your budget allows, look for new or replacement Energy Star-qualified products for energy efficiency.*			
7. Clothes dryer with moisture sensor.			
8. Clothes washer that saves water and energy.			
9. Energy-efficient home-office equipment and electronics.			
10. Replace dangerous, inefficient halogen torchiere lamps with Energy Star-qualified torchieres.			
Low-Cost Home Improvements *These are regular, less expensive things you can do for energy efficiency.*			
1. Replace furnace and air-conditioning filters monthly.			
2. Caulk between window/door frames and walls.			
3. Weatherstrip between doors and frames.			
4. Use window-film kits to improve window energy efficiency (if windows are not already Low-E coated or Energy Star rated).			
5. Insulate hot water heater.			
6. Install motion sensors, dimmers, and timers for indoor and outdoor lighting.			
7. Plant trees to shelter your home from the elements.			
8. Install ceiling or other fans to cut down on air-conditioning costs.			
9. Insulate attic, exterior walls, basement, and crawl spaces.			

No-Cost Energy-Conscious Behaviors	Already in Place	House-hold Goal	Date Achieved
1. Regularly clean reusable furnace and air conditioner filters.			
2. Turn off lights when you leave a room.			
3. Use sunlight for light or heat whenever practical.			
4. Match pot size to burner size and keep the lid on it.			
5. Set hot water heater no higher than 120°F.			
6. Do laundry in cold water.			
7. Use the Energy Star–qualified computer sleep feature.			
8. Turn off electronics when not in use.			
9. Utilize blinds or shades in summer.			
10. Do full loads in dishwashers, clothes washers, and dryers.			
11. Keep your car tuned up and its tires properly inflated.			

Adapted from a brochure provided by Alliance to Save Energy.

Pay a Professional to Perform an Energy Audit ☼ $–$$

If the do-it-yourself approach isn't for you or you don't have the time to spare, then I recommend you hire a professional. Professional audits are often more comprehensive and usually come with a lot of tips and recommendations from the auditor. Contact your local utility or gas company to see if they offer professional home-energy audits, which they will usually conduct for a fee. If not, ask for a referral or look in the telephone directory under "energy." Additionally, the Energy Star Web site has a directory of certified home energy raters.

A typical comprehensive analysis and report would include some or all of the following:

- A room-by-room examination of your home
- An evaluation of past utility bills
- A blower test to determine the general location of air leaks
- An infrared inspection to further locate air leaks and moisture problems
- A list of existing problems like condensation, drafts and air leaks, or clogged filters
- A review of the energy used by your water heater, air conditioner, laundry, refrigerator/freezer, and lighting, as well as your natural gas consumption
- A carbon monoxide check
- Solutions on how to increase your home's energy efficiency

LIFESTYLE ACTION
capture green heat

what you need to know

While you may have energy-efficient appliances, you can also make your home more energy-efficient. Capturing heat from the sun's rays, for instance, will lower the amount of energy you need to buy and will benefit you and your family. After all, the sun is free!

You can harness the power of the sun in very simple ways like letting more sun shine into your home during the winter to heat its interior, or by using a solar-powered calculator. A more costly and complex step would be to install a complete solar system, which collects energy for electricity use, heats water for household use, or heats your pool. Don't write off solar systems! Although they were largely introduced in the 1970s, they have come a long way in being more efficient and cost-effective. There is also financing available. And these days they also look better and can be easily hidden—they can be mounted flush against the roof to look like a skylight and they come in different colors to match the color of your roof. Producing solar power doesn't cause climate change nor does it spew carbon dioxide and other greenhouse gases into the air like the use of oil, coal, or natural gas does. It is one of the simplest and least risky ways we can produce power.

benefits

Capturing heat and the sun's rays can save you money, and because this means purchasing less energy from public utilities, it helps the environment. You can research federal, state, and local tax credits to see if reimbursement is available for the purchase and installation of a solar energy system. Finally, when you sell your home, you can often recoup the entire cost of the system.

how-to's

Cook Smarter for Heat Retention and Energy Efficiency ☺ ∅

Here's a simple tip: Put the lid on your pot when you're cooking on the stove (as long as it does not compromise your dish). Your pot's contents will heat up more quickly because more heat will be captured inside the pan. Otherwise, you're not only heating up your pan and its contents, but also the surrounding air. Additionally, if you are boiling ingredients or water in your pot, reduce the heat to medium or low once you discern a boil, as a roiling boil and a soft boil occur at the exact same temperature. Finally, match pans to burner size; otherwise you will lose heat to the air around the pan.

Wrap Your Water Heater in a Blanket ☺ $

This is an easy insulation technique that helps capture heat you've already paid for and produced so that you will spend (and waste) less. You can purchase and install a water heater blanket for under $25 and start conserving energy today. You don't need a professional to do it. (I'm all for that—more ways to save money!) Wrap the blanket around your water heater and make sure the labels, thermostat access panel, and operational specifications are visible—if not, cut out a "window" so you can see them. The blanket should also have cutouts for the heating coil elements and the combustion air duct. According to the U.S. Department of Energy, you can save between 4 and 9 percent in water heating costs by following through on this simple tip.

>> The average household water-heating bill makes up about 25 percent of a home's energy costs according to the U.S. Department of Energy.

Plant Deciduous Trees ☺ ✚ $–$$

Don't hug a tree, plant one! I have a little deciduous tree (a type of tree that keeps its leaves in the summer but loses them in the winter) in the front of my house. It's brand-new and little more than broomstick-sized, but I was so excited to see the leaves come out in the spring after its planting. In a few more years, that tree will bring us terrific shade in the summer and will allow the sun to shine through during the colder months. Trees also beautify your property and improve your mental health by giving you something lovely and green to look at. Additionally, they improve air quality by absorbing and sequestering carbon dioxide in the air and then turning it back into oxygen. Your property's value may also appreciate by planting trees.

Heat Your Home with Natural Light ☺ ∅

This is simple. Just open your blinds and curtains during the wintertime to bring the sun's rays indoors. The heat from those rays will warm up your home during daylight hours. The added benefit is your reduced need to turn on lightbulbs—again saving you electricity. Plus, the sun's rays prompt our bodies to produce more serotonin, thus boosting our energy.

>> If you want extra insulation for your windows, add some thermal curtains to your window treatments. Leave them open during the day to let in the natural heat and light, but close them at night to use the special fabric as additional insulation against the colder nighttime temperatures.

Upgrade Your Windows ☺ $$–$$$$

When you upgrade your windows to more energy-efficient options, you will trap the heat inside your home more readily (you'll cool your home better, too). One of the cheapest and easiest ways to upgrade your window's insulation is by applying an insulating film directly to the glass—I've done it and found it to be a very cost-effective option. Many of these window-film products come with UV protection, and will shield both your skin and your furniture. You can also upgrade your window treatments to a more insulating type that still gives you light during the day, and/or you can completely replace your windows.

When looking for complete window replacements, one of the most important things to look for are products that carry the Energy Star rating; this will ensure that the product has passed high enough standards to be worth your upgrade money. Energy Star–rated windows will likely be either dual or triple paned for added insulation, have acceptable window ratings for your climate, be built in certain types of frames, and have a Low-E coating to give you more heat or to cool down, depending on your climate. Additionally, Energy Star's Web site lets you search by zip code for manufacturers in your area and tells you the best window options for your climate. I tested this search feature, and since I live in Southern California, I learned that I am in Energy Star's South/Central Climate Zone. This means that certain kinds of coatings and frames will be more energy efficient for my area; in my case, Low-E glass with either wood, vinyl, fiberglass, or composite frames. To recoup some of the initial costs, look for federal or state tax credits offered for installing energy-efficient windows. Your local utility company may also have a credit program that may offer you incentives and rebates.

>> **The U.S. Department of Energy says you can save as much as 50 percent on your heating bills by installing energy-efficient windows in your home. Having adequate insulation in your attic, ceilings, exterior and basement walls, floors, and crawl spaces can knock 30 percent of your home energy bill.**

the lowdown on low-e

Low-E (or low-emissivity) glass has been coated with a virtually invisible, superthin metallic glaze for purposes of energy-efficiency. This coating is either already encased in the window's glass panes by the manufacturer, or included in window film that either you or a professional add to the window. Low-E glass also cuts down on UV light, which can fade carpets, fabric, and furniture—and reducing UV light also helps to protect your skin and eyes. Brand-new Low-E windows cost 10 to 15 percent more than regular new windows, but according to the Department of Energy, they will reduce your energy costs by as much as 30 to 50 percent—a real money saver!

There are also other quality window films available that are not labeled Low-E but offer tremendous energy-efficiency, protect from harmful UV rays, and come with energy rebates. They typically last ten to fifteen years (or longer) without peeling and can recoup their costs within a year, allowing you to save for the day when you can purchase new windows. Some of these films are remarkably clear, with virtually no reflectivity, and allow a fabulous clear view of the outdoors. You want to avoid reflective film; in my opinion, it's not attractive. Plus, it can be deceptive and harmful to birds, which could fly into your windows because they see the sky's reflection.

3M >> (www.3m.com) Clear-window, energy-saving window film—dealer-installed only

GILA FILMS >> (www.gilafilms.com) Do-it-yourself Low-E window film that offers excellent, immediate heat reduction

SOLAR GARD >> (www.solargard.com) Window films with Low-E and heat control—dealer-installed only

Fill In Cracks ☺ $-$$
Sealing up air leaks is relatively easy to do. You can use caulk, weather-stripping, spray foam, or duct sealant for ducts (also called duct mastic).

If your sealant will remain visible, make sure it is aesthetically pleasing or can be painted over. Most air drafts are easy to find around windows because you can feel the cool or warm air seeping into your home, but there are other places to look for air leaks and drafts, including:

- Dryer vent
- Outdoor electrical outlets
- Door frames
- Attic hatch
- Recessed lighting fixtures
- Bathroom fan vents
- Plumbing stack vents
- Kitchen fan vents
- Outdoor faucets
- Exposed ducts in attics, basements, crawl spaces, and garages

how to caulk your windows

If you have drafts coming in through the sides of your windows, you should look for cracks in the seals between the outside wall and the window frame. You can purchase caulk from your local hardware store for under $10 and fill in these cracks for more energy-efficiency and insulation. Some caulk requires a caulking gun, which acts as leverage to push the caulk through the tip. Caulk has the consistency of glue, so you can smooth it out with your finger and easily clean up mistakes, but once it dries it can be difficult to remove. Make sure you've applied it only where you want to fill in the cracks, and consider paintable caulk if you want to perform some paint touch-ups after your crack is repaired.

>> **Close the damper on your fireplace when you don't have a fire burning.** According to the California Energy Commission, an open damper can let 8 percent of heat escape through your chimney, not to mention cool air escaping during the summer months. If you are going to burn a fire for heat, choose eco-friendly logs

(continued)

over traditional wood. Some are man-made logs that burn longer, produce fewer emissions, and are made out of nontoxic, recycled materials.

JAVA-LOG >> (www.java-log.com) Fire logs made from recycled spent coffee grounds and all-natural vegetable wax—100 percent renewable resources—that produce 70–80 percent less emissions than wood

PINE MOUNTAIN LOGS >> (www.pinemountainbrands.com) Clean-burning fire logs

fresh is in

For most older homes, sealing up air drafts is energy-wise. However, if you have a newer home or even a well-sealed older home, you may want to get the advice of a home energy professional, who has the ability to detect how much actual air leakage and fresh air you have in your home. According to the EPA, we need fresh air in our homes for our family's health as much as we need our homes to be insulated—especially since we are spending up to 90 percent of our time indoors. If you're in a climate or season of the year that doesn't allow you to regularly open up your windows and doors to get fresh air, then home air pollutants, mold, and carbon monoxide can accumulate to risky levels. In fact, according to the Environmental Protection Agency, indoor air is likely to be four to five times worse than outdoor air due to lack of ventilation. And the American College of Allergy, Asthma and Immunology states that 50 percent of all illnesses are either caused or aggravated by polluted indoor air.

For solutions other than opening your windows and doors, you'll need mechanical ways to ventilate your air. At the very least, your kitchen and bathroom exhaust fans can pull air out of your home and push it to the outdoors—this offers some exhaust ventilation.

But you can also talk to a contractor about installing a supply and exhaust ventilation system that brings in fresh outdoor air and exhausts old indoor air. Most heating and cooling systems do not provide supply and exhaust ventilation but rather recirculate the same air over and over.

Consider installing a whole-home air purifier onto your central air system for the most effective and safest way of cleaning up both recirculating and fresh air in your home. Or, you could buy a portable air purifier—the HEPA air purifiers are the best—just make sure there are no ozone emissions. Check with Energy Star for product options.

All air cleaners and purifiers should list the clean air delivery rate so that you can comparison shop and know their true effectiveness—clean air delivery rates range from 10 to 1,200, with the highest number being the best. And whole-house air cleaners will have a higher clean air delivery rate than portable air cleaners.

Here are other ways you can keep your indoor air fresh and clean:

- Reduce your fireplace usage.
- If it's possible, have your pet stay outdoors to reduce pet dander.
- Leave fireplace logs outside until you're ready to use them, as they can contain mold.
- Vacuum with a HEPA-filter vacuum (see ideas in the cleaning section).
- Open the windows on a regular basis to get fresh air circulation.
- Use your stove fan when cooking to ventilate smoke outdoors.
- Upgrade your lights to reduce emissions. (When you reduce your electrical use with more efficient lights, you reduce greenhouse gas emissions by using less emission-producing electricity and requiring fewer lightbulb replacements.)
- Change out the air filters for your central ventilation unit—on average, once a month.
- Clean reusable furnace and air conditioner filters every month during the heating and cooling seasons.
- Add indoor plants to help clean the air.

- Reduce air freshener usage, which can add chemicals to your air.
- Burn no-soot candles so that your air doesn't become polluted from traditional candles made with paraffin and petroleum; soy candles are usually soot and toxin free.

ELECTROLUX >> (www.electrolux.com) Hood ventilation for your kitchen

BROAN >> (www.broan.com) Quality Energy Star–rated home-ventilation systems

TRANE >> (www.trane.com) Sells a high-quality whole-house air cleaner, as well as a whole-house ventilation system that exhausts stale indoor air and brings in fresh air

---

Upgrade Your Doors ☺ $–$$$$

There are a number of ways you can upgrade your doors to be more energy efficient and keep heated or cooled air from escaping your home. One of the easiest and least expensive ways is by installing weather-stripping insulation around your doors. You can do it yourself and stripping is readily available at your local hardware store. If your door already has weatherstripping, consider replacing it if it looks worn. Additionally, you can add a door sweep to further insulate.

A more expensive option is replacing your door. Many of the newest versions are highly energy efficient, preferably measured and installed by a professional so that its quality is maintained. Some newer doors are manufactured with a magnetic strip that serves as weatherstripping. If you purchase doors with windows in them or doors that are all glass, pay attention to energy-efficient options because glass does not insulate as well as a solid door. You can look for Energy Star ratings, Low-E coatings, and possibly a NFRC label to help you make the most energy-efficient choice of windowed doors.

Doors will likely come with an R-value rating between R-1 and R-7. A higher R-value means the door has better insulation. Remember to look for federal tax credits for upgrading your door.

all about nfrc

Besides looking for Energy Star–rated doors and windows, you can make additional comparisons of your purchases by utilizing the labeling system of the National Fenestration Rating Council, or NFRC (www .nrfc.org). This independent, nonprofit organization rates and compares the energy and performance features of windows, doors, and skylights. The NFRC label gives performance ratings in four categories—all of which are helpful to consumers but are technical and require that you know what you're looking for. A sample NFRC window label is provided here. NFRC door labels usually only carry the U-Factor and SHGC ratings.

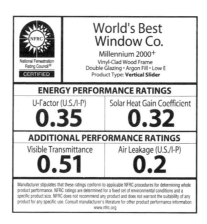

U-Factor (Look for a Lower Number)

The U-Factor measures how well a window, door, or skylight insulates. The lower the U-Factor, the better the window or door insulates. U-Factor ratings generally fall between 0.20 and 1.25. Energy Star's Web site can help you find the ideal U-Factor for your region.

Solar Heat Gain Coefficient (Look for a Lower Number)

The Solar Heat Gain Coefficient (SHGC) measures how well a window, door, or skylight blocks heat emitted by the sun. This is especially important if you live in a hot, sunny area and don't want to add heat to your home. The SHGC is expressed as a number between zero and one. The lower the SHGC, the less heat will be transmitted into your home. Energy Star's Web site can help you find the ideal SHGC for your geographic area.

Visible Transmittance (Look for a Higher Number)

Visible Transmittance (VT) measures how much light comes through your window or skylight. VT is expressed as a number between zero and one. The higher the VT, the more light you see and the better your view of the outdoors.

Air Leakage* (Look for a Lower Number)

Air Leakage (AL) measures the rate at which air passes through cracks in the window or skylight assembly. You can lose and gain heat through these cracks, so the Air Leakage rating is a further indication of insulation. The lower the AL rating, the less air will pass through cracks in the window assembly. In general, look for windows with an AL of 0.30 or lower.

Condensation Resistance* (Look for a Higher Number)

Condensation Resistance (CR) is often not included on the NFRC label and was not included on this sample label. However, if you see it, know that the rating measures the ability of a product to resist the formation of condensation on the interior surface of that product. You don't want condensation on your window because not only does it reduce the ability to see out, but it also can cause gradual water damage to curtains, walls, carpets, and even the windows itself. The higher the CR rating, the better that product is at resisting condensation formation. CR is expressed as a number between 0 and 100.

---

*This rating is optional and manufacturers can choose not to include it.

opening up about wood and fiberglass

Although a lot of people want a traditional wood door for their home, some might be surprised to know that today's high-quality fiberglass doors look exactly the same as a wood door. The quality and feel is usually the same as wood, but fiberglass lasts much longer and provides up to five times the insulation. Fiberglass doors are resistant to weather, termites, warping and cracking; contain energy-efficient cores; and retain their original look with virtually no maintenance.

The downside is fiberglass doors cannot be recycled, only reused (on another door frame, for example). While wood doors can be recycled, they don't have the insulating properties, savings on maintenance, or lasting use that fiberglass doors do. Since there are pros and cons with both wood and fiberglass doors, make the choice that will last the longest.

THERMA-TRU DOORS >> (www.thermatru.com) Manufactures Energy Star-rated, high-quality, beautiful doors, including fiberglass—and uses a variety of recycled products in its doors, including recycled wood chips, diapers, and plastic bottles.

JELD-WEN >> (www.jeld-wen.com) Sells high-quality doors and windows that are energy efficient. Jeld-Wen is also an Energy Star partner. The company's windows come standard with Low-E. And for overall green living, Jeld-Wen has several products that use recycled content and use less toxic manufacturing processes (to reduce volatile organic compounds, or VOCs—toxic gases that can pollute your air). It also has manufacturing sites across the United States, which means the company uses less fuel for transportation. The company is also committed to sustainable forestry.

Upgrade Your Home's Wall and Ceiling Insulation ☺ $$$–$$$$

You can improve the retention of heat and cold in your home by improving your wall and ceiling insulation. Ideally, your home already has wall insulation, especially if you live in a colder climate, because tearing down walls and adding insulation is a major investment, not to mention a hassle. Contact a professional for that task and ask about spray-in options so that you don't have to tear down walls.

A much simpler thing you can do to improve your home's energy efficiency is adding more insulation to your attic. If you are able to stick an ordinary ruler into your attic's current insulation and can still see the top of the ruler, you would be wise to consider adding more insulation. An ideal level in the attic would be twelve to fifteen inches of insulation. All it requires, in many cases, is the contractor blowing another layer of insulation up into the attic, and this can be done in less than an hour. Other methods include laying additional insulation batting over the existing insulation, which you can do yourself. Make sure your recessed lighting and exhaust fans are *not* covered up by this insulation.

When considering the type of insulation to be installed or added into your home, look at the R-value. A higher R-value means the insulation is more insulating. For homes in cooler climates where heat retention is critical, the ideal R-value would be around R-49 for ceiling insulation. For warmer climates, it would be approximately R-38 for ceiling insulation. A complete insulation guide with recommended R-values is available at www .energystar.gov.

ICYNENE >> (www.icynene.com) Energy Star–rated household insulation that can also be used to easily fill walls in older homes without taking down existing structures or walls.

Install a Solar Water Heating System for Your Household Water Use and/or Your Pool ☺ $$$$

There's another way you can turn heat from the sun into something you need. A solar water heating system gets heat from a solar panel collector on your rooftop and then feeds the heat collected to your water heater or to an insulated storage tank. In the case of heating your pool water, the pool's filtration pump circulates the water through the collector to capture the heat and returns that warmed water back into your pool.

The Department of Energy has a consumer's guide that explains, in detail, the difference between the various solar water heating systems; the key is to do your own research before you make a selection. Also, check your local building code requirements to make sure that your system would be to code.

Although a solar water heating system can cost you more to purchase and install than a conventional electric water heater, over the long term it can save you money—as much as 50 to 80 percent on your water heating bills, according to the Department of Energy. If a family stays in the same house for many years, they will save money over the long term simply because of the amount of hot water a family uses. Additionally, the more sun you have in your geographic area, the more heat you'll be able to produce for free and, since the sun doesn't hike rates, you've protected yourself from market fluctuations.

You should also look for any rebates that might be offered by your state or local municipality, or look for a federal government tax credit. Your contractor might also know of rebates or credits to apply for.

>> In China, 62 percent of the population heats its water through solar systems.

RHEEM: >> Solar water heaters with information found at www.smarterhotwater.com.

Capture Heat in Your Pool with a Solar Cover ☺ ☼ $-$$$

Want an easy way to heat your pool? Try a solar pool cover, which will help attract and trap the heat from the sun's rays so you can reduce your need for a pool heater. You'll save yourself money and use less energy. You can also achieve up to a 15 percent temperature rise from the sun alone when using a solar pool cover, which can be great news for you if you live in a colder climate. Not only do you have this energy benefit, but the cover also protects your pool's water from debris and keeps it cleaner. This, in turn, saves you time and energy if you regularly run an automatic pool vacuum or cleaner. Furthermore, a quality solar cover can cut water evaporation by up to 95 percent. Save some time by investing in a reel, which can easily take the cover off and on, and keeps it in great condition.

Heat Your Home with a Solar Space Heating System ☺ $$$$

While solar water heating is relatively straightforward, heating your entire home with solar energy generally requires a larger and more complex system. Such a system can supply your home with 40–60 percent of your space-heating needs if you get enough sunlight. This "if" part is important, because typically there is less sunlight in the winter, which is when you need the heat the most.

To find out if the savings will be worth it, you'll need to average in the savings versus the cost and calculate how many years will pass before you see a payoff. Many solar space heating vendors have a savings calculator which takes into consideration where you live in determining how much sun, on average, you are apt to receive during the year and how much savings that will translate to. Depending on where you live, you may find that a more cost-effective way to heat your home is through better insulation and capturing the sun's heat through your windows.

Utilize Solar Power ☺ $$$$

You have likely used solar power many, many times in your life without realizing it. The perfect example is a solar-powered calculator that uses clean energy from a light source or the sun—once the calculator is purchased you never need to pay another dime to keep it working. This solar-power technology is called photovoltaics (or PV) and can also be found in:

- Battery chargers
- Radios
- Lamps
- Garden lights
- Flashlights

You can install solar panels—also known as a PV system—on your property or on your roof to produce clean energy from the sun. I did several calculations of what it would cost me to install a PV system on my home in Southern California. I learned it would provide me with approximately 50–70 percent of my electrical needs and would take me about eleven years to break even after the installation. My home is in a sunny area of the United States and has an electric bill of more than $75 per month. If I were to install a PV system, I would likely be able to recoup at least a third to half of the initial cost when I sell my home because of the appreciation value such a system gives the home. And even before I sell, I would be able to garner an estimated $9,720 utility rebate and a federal tax credit of $2,000. But the important bottom line I learned is that PV is likely a long-term investment, no matter the future savings or the fact that it is one of the cleanest sources of energy.

If you are interested in a solar system, you need to carefully review numbers given to you from three or more solar system providers. Make sure those providers are including any additional costs in their proposals, such as preparation of your roof for the installation, or additional options like power storage. And be sure you look into utility rebates and tax credits/deductions. Financing is also available, and leasing options are emerging as a possibility as well. The good news is that by installing a PV system, you can safeguard your family from future energy price hikes, reduce your electrical bills, and make an environmental impact the equivalent of planting two acres of trees per year.

Cook Using the Sun ☺ $$

If you camp, enjoy picnics, like to cook outdoors, or want to make sure you have a way to cook in the event of a power failure, consider buying a solar oven. With it, you don't need anything else besides a sunny day to bake, boil, or steam food. You won't need gas or briquettes, and there are no greenhouse gases or waste emitted, which is great news for the environment, your air, and your pocketbook. Some solar ovens come with a power source hookup, so you can enjoy added flexibility and more temperature control when you need it; these hybrid versions also have electric power kick in when the sun is going in and out of clouds.

is solar power worth it?

No matter your climate, you can take advantage of solar power technologies. Just to compare, if you live in a state with a high number of per-day sun hours, you can generate up to 8.5 kilowatt-hours (kWh) per day in electricity for your home's use. If you compare that with the states that are the northernmost and get the least amount of sun, you're still going to generate an average of 5.0 kWh per day in electricity from your solar system. So, considering that the average home uses about 29 kWh per day, you could be getting almost a third of your energy per day for free if you had a solar system—not to mention that the sun's energy doesn't cost more as time goes by, so you are also insulated from rising energy costs.

>> While the overall housing market in California cooled in 2007, one exception was homes with solar power, which outsold nonsolar homes.

look for solar system ratings

As you can tell, I am a big fan of ratings systems, certifications, and licenses. They are the most reliable way to quickly ascertain quality levels. For solar systems that produce electricity for your home, the Florida Solar Energy Center (FSEC; www.floridaenergycenter.org) certifies PV models and systems and lists them on its Web site. Certification means that the FSEC has tested the product for reliability, safety, and overall quality. The certification provides you with additional manufacturer information about the product, the expected power output, and installer information so your PV system will meet building codes. Although there is no standard ratings system for comparing the quality of PV models and systems, a certification is a solid benchmark you can use when selecting a contractor. If the PV system being proposed by your contractor is not certified by the FSEC, then it should be certified by some other verifiable, unbiased organization—perhaps another state's agency that deals with solar energy.

questions to ask a solar panel expert

It's always smart to get referrals when you are hiring a contractor, and you want to screen solar system specialists before purchasing their services. Good questions to ask:

- *What kind of experience does your company have in installing and maintaining solar water heating systems?* Do your research ahead of time to know what kind of system you would like to purchase so that you can gauge the knowledge and experience of the professional.
- *How many years of experience do you and your business have?* It is important that the company has a solid list of references and successful projects completed.
- *Are you licensed or certified?* Many states license or certify their contractors. It is always best to look for a licensed or certified contractor so you have recourse if the job goes bad. You should confirm this licensing or certification with your state board and check if there are any complaints on file. You can also check with the Better Business Bureau (www.bbb .org).

SOLARWORLD >> (www.solarworld-usa.com) High-quality solar power modules/systems backed by a twenty-five-year warranty. The company includes recycling efforts in both production of the modules and the product's end of life.

BP SOLAR >> (www.bpsolar.us) Sells solar solutions for homes, businesses, and builders. A solar savings calculator can be found on the site, and the company's solar systems are available through Home Depot.

LIFESTYLE ACTION

cool off more efficiently

what you need to know

As much as we love and need the sun, it can really heat up our homes in the summer months, or year-round in warmer climates. And if global warming continues, many areas of the country are going to be warmer than ever, which can lead to higher costs for cooling down. The good news is there are many eco-friendly things you can do to head off undesired heat. Ideally, your daytime indoor temperature should be a comfort level of somewhere between 74 and 80°F. At nighttime, it should be lower, as most people sleep better when the indoor temperature is around 60–65°F. Consider combining efficient air-conditioning with my tips and tricks to gain maximum monetary and energy savings by achieving your home's ideal temperature.

summer temps

Most utility companies recommend that you set your summer thermostat temperature to no lower than 76 degrees in the summertime to save energy. You might be able to set it higher, at 78 or 79, if you take advantage of fans because they can make you feel up to five degrees cooler. Consider setting the temperature to 85 degrees when you are away from home, as long as food and electronics will not be damaged.

benefits

Save money and keep your home cooler by integrating energy-saving and eco-friendly practices into your lifestyle.

how-to's

Plant Trees to Shade Your Home ☺ ✚ $–$$$$
One of the best things you can do for your family, the environment, your comfort, and your property's value is to strategically plant trees around your home. Your south-, east-, and west-facing windows will be the most vulnerable to summer heat and can benefit the most from

trees that produce shade during the warmest parts of the year. Trees can help reduce your need for air-conditioning by as much as 30 percent, increase your property's value by 15 percent or more, improve the air you breathe, and impart natural beauty that benefits your mental health. The cost of planting trees depends on the type of tree you are buying and how old it is. Older trees will cost you more and be more difficult to plant because of their size and weight. If you are going to plant bigger, more mature trees, it is advised that you hire the nursery or a professional landscaper to do the preparation and planting for you. They will also help you determine if you have proper irrigation in place. Many communities have tree-planting programs that offer free or discounted trees to residents who are willing to properly take care of them. Plant deciduous trees if you want the added benefit of sunshine heat to warm up your home in the wintertime. Additionally, when a whole neighborhood plants lots of trees, it has a combination effect and cools down the entire neighborhood—not just your home. According to the Arbor Day Foundation (www.arborday .org), shade trees that are near your home can cut cooling costs by 15–35 percent. Wildlife are also served by trees, especially those that flower and produce fruit or nuts. This helps to provide a healthy ecosystem for bees, birds, and other wildlife. And your family can also benefit by having fruit and nut trees by enjoying low-cost produce that you can also grow organically, protecting you from food cost increases and food safety risks.

>> **Trees remove carbon dioxide from the air and help fight global warming.**

Shade from the Inside with Effective Window Treatments ☺ $–$$$$

Your window treatments can provide another layer of insulation against the elements—either by keeping in the heat on cold days or by blocking out the heat on hot days. High-quality window treatments will also help you block harmful UV rays. When I lived in Phoenix for several years, we had honeycomb shades on the windows that got the most sun. They really help keep the heat level down. Most manufacturers display the features and benefits of their window treatments on their Web sites and in their product showrooms at large hardware stores and design centers. Some of the treatments to consider include:

- Honeycomb/cellular horizontal fabric shades have air pockets that provide additional insulation; light-filtering options also provide needed daytime light.
- Woven shades made with sustainable materials like bamboo, reeds, or grasses.
- Roman fabric shades.
- Faux wood shutters, which won't warp or fade with the sun.
- Solar roller shades are like sunglasses for your windows, and can still offer you an outside view with filtered daylight (but may not provide you with the higher insulating value of other window treatments).
- Drapes and curtains. Most can offer you some solar protection, and those that can are labeled "thermal" or "insulated." However, other than insulating at night against the cold, there are much better alternatives for daytime applications that both let the natural light in as well as provide you the insulating value you desire during both hot and cold seasons.

HUNTER DOUGLAS >> (www.hunterdouglas.com) Leader in honeycomb shades and many other window coverings; has a designer fabric option which contains no PVC, no emissions, and is recyclable (see page 163 for more information on PVC).

SPRINGS WINDOW FASHIONS (BALI, GRABER, AND NANIK BRANDS) >> (www.springswindowfashions.com) Solar shades that block up to 95 percent of heat, have UV protection, and low VOC emissions.

Shade from the Outside with Special Screens, Shades, and Awnings ☺ $-$$$$

Special fiberglass screens, which serve the traditional function of keeping out the bugs, also block more than 80 percent of the sun's heat before it even hits the glass. Keep in mind that they are darker looking on the outside of your home—and function as privacy screens—even though your inside view isn't compromised.

You can also add an outdoor shade or awning. Some of these require professional installation, but they will offer additional shade without blocking your view of the outdoors.

PHIFER >> (www.phifer.com) Do-it-yourself solar exterior screens and interior solar shading products.

Open Your Windows at Night ☺ ∅

I love opening the windows at night. It allows any heat that built up during the day to escape, and I can then cool off my house for free. I live in California where the nights are generally cool. If you live in an area that similarly cools off at night during the summer, then open up your windows once the sun goes down (provided you have screens to block out the bugs). Your home and family need the fresh air circulation and ventilation. If you struggle with allergies, this strategy may not be your best option; otherwise, it's the most natural way to enjoy cool, fresh air.

Install and Use Ceiling Fans Throughout Your Home ☺ $-$$$$

I've always loved ceiling fans. They cool a room and free up your air-conditioning usage. Energy Star-rated ceiling fans are the most energy efficient and can move air 20 percent more effectively than other models.

Ceiling fans are more useful than traditional floor fans because they are more effective at circulating the air in the room and can help you set a higher thermostat temperature, allowing you to feel about four or five degrees cooler when the fan is running. The fans also increase your personal evaporation rate which cools you off—basically, the circulating air evaporates the small beads of sweat on your skin which gives a windchill-type cooling effect, just as if there were a cool breeze in the air. A larger ceiling fan will provide you more cooling benefit than a smaller fan, but read the box labels or product specifications carefully and match the size of the fan to the size of the room.

Running an energy-efficient fan is a lot cheaper than running your central air-conditioning unit. A ceiling fan is not an item you want to cut costs on; many of the more expensive ones really do offer added benefits in terms of quality materials and quiet use.

Because there's no benefit to the ceiling fan being on when you're not around, only run it when you are in the room. Be sure to follow the operating instructions—one blade rotation gives a cooling effect by blowing the air downward, and the other direction is for wintertime use as it pushes hot air up into the ceiling and down toward the walls to circulate it through the room. Also, be sure that your computer equipment and electronics will not be affected by a higher thermostat setting, as a ceiling fan will not reduce the temperature of those items. For safety reasons, do not install a ceiling fan in a room with a ceiling that is less than eight feet high, with blades no closer than eight inches from the ceiling and eighteen inches from the walls.

HUNTER >> (www.hunterfan.com) Energy Star–rated, high-quality fans.

SEA GULL LIGHTING >> (www.seagulllighting.com) Ceiling fans with Energy Star rating.

Use Traditional Fans to Cool Off ☺ $-$$

If the cost of ceiling fans is too prohibitive, or if your living situation doesn't allow for one, floor fans are a great alternative cool-off option. Again, look for the Energy Star logo on the product—this will ensure that you have the most efficient model. On the comfort side, it is best to find a fan that is as quiet as possible. Granted, this can be hard to determine until you buy it, so make sure the store has a liberal return policy.

Don't Leave the Refrigerator or Freezer Open ☺

It takes a lot of energy to cool down the interior of your fridge and freezer, and every time you open those doors a whole lot of cold air gets out. Train your family (and yourself!) to not stand for long periods of time in front of an open refrigerator or freezer. And close the doors in between restocking when you put away your groceries.

Don't Put Your Freezer or Refrigerator in the Garage ☺

While it may be tempting to free up some space, unless you have an insulated garage with the temperature regulated just like inside your home or if you live in a cool climate, don't put your freezer or a second refrigerator in the garage. It will simply cost too much to keep it cold. The one exception is if you don't use your freezer in the summer and can keep it turned off.

Schedule Heat-Generating Activities for the Evening ☺ ∅

Some activities such as oven or stove-top cooking, or using the dishwasher or dryer, generate extra heat. During the warmest months of the year, consider cooking with less indoor heat by using a slow cooker, a microwave, or an outside grill or solar oven. Wait until evening to use the dishwasher or dryer and you'll reduce the heat in your home during the daytime hours. Some dishwashers have a handy timer feature that allows you to set a washing time (perfect for late-in-the-evening dish washings). Ask your utility company if they offer a time-of-use discount—this means that your utility would charge you different rates for different times of the day; during peak times, you would be charged more.

Install a Heat Pump ☺ $$$$

Why is "heat pump" in this "cool off" section? Don't let the name fool you. This efficient home comfort system is basically a central air-conditioning unit that *also* heats your home during cold weather. There are three kinds of heat pumps in the marketplace to choose from—air, ground, and water.

• An *air-source* heat pump extracts heat from the air and brings it into your home to heat it in the winter and releases heat from your home back into the outside air to cool your home in the summer. And, yes, this works in cold weather for heating your home because in most places in the United States, there is still heat to be found in the air even in cold weather.

• A *geothermal or ground-source* heat pump extracts heat from the earth around your property to heat your home, and, conversely, sinks heat from the inside of your home back into the earth to cool off your home. It is easier to find heat in the earth, rather than in the air, during cold winter months because beyond a few feet, the earth stays a constant temperature even during the winter. The Environmental Protection Agency (EPA) says that geothermal heat pumps are the most energy-efficient, environmentally clean, and cost-effective option for space heating. In fact, the EPA found that geothermal heat pumps reduce energy consumption and emissions by over 40 percent compared to air-source heat pumps, and by over 70 percent compared to traditional electric heating and cooling systems (such as traditional air conditioners and furnaces).

• A *water-source* heat pump extracts heat from below-ground aquifers, a nearby water source, or a boiler unit / cooling tower to heat your home; for cooling off your home, it expels heat to those same sources. Again, because the technology is going below ground and not into the air, it is easier to find heat in the winter months.

A heat pump replaces your furnace *and* your air conditioner, so consider this an efficient upgrade. It can heat your water, as well, if you choose that option. When selecting a heat pump, make sure the heat pump has the Energy Star rating. Also, look for and compare three other ratings: SEER, HSPF, and EER ratings. (See pages 32–33 for definitions.) You want the highest numbers possible. Like other big-ticket appliances, heat pumps are an investment that has the greatest guarantee of paying for itself if you are going to be living in your residence for several more years. A reputable contractor or the product's manufacturer should be able to provide you with an analysis of your investment to tell you when you can project to break even and what other cost savings the unit will provide you. Additionally, the contractor or the manufacturer should know what rebates or tax incentives are available in your area to help off-set the cost of a new heat pump.

Heat pumps can be up to three times more energy efficient at heat-ing your water than your conventional water heater. This is because a heat pump just moves heat that already exists in nature to heat your wa-ter. But conventional units have to make heat with electricity—this uses more energy and, therefore, is more expensive.

CARRIER >> (www.carrier.com) Complete line of energy-efficient heat pumps, ventilation, and air-conditioning products.

CLIMATEMASTER >> (www.climatemaster.com) Geothermal heat pumps.

FHP MANUFACTURING >> (www.fhp-mfg.com) Geothermal and water-source heat pumps.

GOODMAN >> (www.goodmanmfg.com) Air-source heat pumps and high-SEER-rated air-conditioning systems.

TRANE >> (www.trane.com) Air-source heat pumps and high-SEER-rated air conditioners.

Upgrade Your AC or Evaporative Cooler Unit ☺ $$$–$$$$

If it's time to upgrade your air conditioner or evaporative cooler (some-times called a swamp cooler), first and foremost, consider a heat pump. If that's not an option and you live in a dry, hot climate, consider an evaporative cooler with a high CFM rating, which represents the cubic feet per minute of air it delivers into a home.

An evaporative cooler in a dry climate is more efficient than an air-conditioning unit; in fact, the California Energy Commission says that evaporative coolers can use 75 percent less energy than air-conditioning. These coolers are also much less expensive to install—in many cases almost half the cost of an AC unit—and some are powered solely by solar. While an air-conditioning unit recirculates the same air over and over, evaporative coolers bring in fresh air, which is a lot healthier. Some evaporative coolers continuously use water as well, so if you have limited water supplies in your area, you may decide against an evaporative cooler. You'll have to make a judgment call based on your circumstance and area.

If you choose an air conditioner over a heat pump or evaporative cooler, look for not only the Energy Star rating but also the highest SEER and EER ratings you can find. Research whether your state, city, or local public utility offers rebates for upgrading your air conditioner or evaporative cooler to more energy-efficient models. Make sure that the company you hire to install your new evaporative cooler or AC unit has helped you: (1) calculate the square footage to be cooled and recommended a unit that will cool that much square footage, and (2) is selling you the right size for your duct system. If you're not sure, contact the manufacturer before you buy to double-check.

what's going on with seer, hspf, eer, and cfm?

When you buy an air conditioner, evaporative cooler, or a heat pump, you should not only look for the Energy Star logo but also the SEER, HSPF, and EER ratings. Here's what to look for with each type of product.

SEER stands for Seasonal Energy Efficiency Ratio. This is the cooling rating found on heat pumps and air-conditioning units that describes how well the product works over an entire season. *The higher the SEER rating, the more efficient it is.* In order to get an Energy Star rating, both air-source heat pumps and air conditioners must have a *SEER rating greater than or equal to fourteen.*

EER stands for Energy Efficiency Ratio. This rating is a measure of how efficiently a cooling system will operate when the outdoor temperature is at a specific level, usually 95°F. *The higher the EER rating, the more efficient the unit.* For both air conditioners and heat pumps, the Energy Star rating is given to products that have an EER rating *greater than or equal to 11.5 EER for split systems and 11 EER for single-package equipment.* The EER rating is most important when considering geothermal heat pumps; the minimum EER rating for Energy Star approval is 14.1–16.2 EER (depending on the system type).

While EER and SEER appear to be the same thing, they aren't because they give numbers for different modes: SEER is for *overall system efficiency throughout the entire season* and EER is for the system's *energy efficiency at peak cooling operations.* Look for higher numbers for both EER and SEER to help you compare products and discern the most efficient models.

HSPF stands for the Heating Season Performance Factor and is found on air-source heat pump units because they generate both hot and cold air. The HSPF number is a measure of the air-source heat pump's efficiency over the entire season, similar to what SEER is for cooling efficiency. You want to look for the *highest HSPF rating.* The Energy Star rating is given to air-source heat pumps with a HSPH rating that is *greater than or equal to 8.2 HSPF for split systems and 8.0 HSPF for single-package systems.*

CFM stands for cubic feet per minute and is found on evaporative coolers. It measures how much cubic feet of air per minute is delivered into your home—basically, the power of the cooler unit. You want to look for evaporative coolers with *higher CFM ratings.*

Upgrade Your Insulation ☺ $–$$$$

In the Capture Green Heat section (page 6), I've outlined a number of ways you can insulate your home for the greatest energy efficiency. Refer to that section for ideas and tips that are as good for maintaining heat in the winter as keeping your home cool in the summer.

earth-wise water and lighting: using elements the eco-friendly way

Can you imagine what would happen if your family spent a day in your house without lights or water? Mayhem (and possibly strange smells after sports practice)! Water and light have long been essential to our survival, but now that they are both readily available in our homes, we have a tendency to go overboard. Don't worry, you don't have to return to the prairie to do right by Mother Earth when it comes to this pair. Check out the tips in this section and revolutionize the way these elements are used in your home.

LIFESTYLE ACTION

light up with a conscience

what you need to know

Our bodies need light; it regulates our sleep patterns and our energy levels, and the right lighting provides happiness and comfort as we enjoy and decorate our homes. Lighting used to be a simple 60-watt commodity—in fact, the traditional incandescent lightbulb that produces both heat and light (and uses a lot of electricity to do it) has been around since the 1880s. In recent years, millions in research, development, and marketing dollars have been poured into creating new types of home lighting. A trip to a big-box hardware store like Home Depot will have you swimming in hundreds of lighting options. It takes a conscious consumer armed with a bit of knowledge to seek out the type of lighting right for the earth and health.

benefits

Choosing eco-friendly lighting saves you money and is better for the environment and your family's health.

how-to's

Turn the Lights On Only When You Need Them ☺

If there is one easy tip that remains evergreen for being kind to the earth and your pocketbook, it is to turn off your lights when you don't need them.

Get Your Light from the Sun ☺ ✚ ∅-$$$$

Let the sun shine in! It's the greenest option around. On average, we spend almost 90 percent of our time indoors, and during much of that time we are surrounded by lighting that is not very bright. However, sunshine—natural daylight—has been proven to be critical to our everyday health. Of course you want your skin and eyes to be protected from UV rays, but a regular dose of sunlight each day, especially in the morning, keeps you healthy and helps you to avoid seasonal affective disorder. You actually *need* the bright light of sunshine—especially outdoors where it is unshaded—to boost your energy. In fact, sunlight increases the presence of a chemical in our brains called serotonin that (among other benefits) helps us feel good and energetic, lifts our spirits, and improves our thinking and alertness.

Although outdoor light is the best, you can increase the amount of sunshine in your home by opening your blinds and window shades. You can also install new-generation skylighting, which brings in natural daylight without the harmful UV rays and added heat. Many skylights feature options like clear views, light diffusers, dimmers, and ventilation. Look for skylighting that has an Energy Star rating.

Another option is to simulate sunlight through quality daylight lights. Bright-white LED lights are the closest replica of natural sunshine and are often used in new-generation portable light boxes to help people overcome seasonal affective disorder.

SOLATUBE >> (www.solatube.com) Excellent new-generation tubular skylights with an Energy Star rating.

TAM SKYLIGHTS >> (www.tamskylights.com) Energy Star–rated skylights, also available with Low-E and with the ability to open up (to improve ventilation).

Upgrade Your Lightbulbs to Save Electricity and Reduce Waste ☺ ✿ $–$$

Most of us grew up with the traditional incandescent lightbulb as the only kind of lightbulb in the house, but now those bulbs are about to go the way of the typewriter because of their inefficiency. These bulbs are power hungry and produce a lot of unwanted heat, so look for new lighting options to brighten your home; save time, money, and energy; and help the environment.

Currently, the best and most widely distributed bulbs for energy efficiency are Energy Star–rated compact fluorescent lamps (CFLs). CFLs are available in many shapes and types wherever incandescent bulbs are sold. Yes, they will cost more than traditional bulbs, but they last up to ten times longer and produce very little heat. Don't forget to upgrade your outdoor lights as well, as they're often left on all night. Replacing bulbs throughout your house will result in energy savings. Also, look for rebates from your utility company for upgrading your lighting to more efficient options. Light-emitting diode lights (LEDs) are another up-and-coming lighting alternative with even more energy advantages than CFLs, but they haven't done well at illuminating an entire room like CFLs have. Hopefully, technology will overcome this issue, as LEDs pose less environmental hazards than CFLs and are excellent at replicating the sun's natural light.

Learn How to Read a Lightbulb's Label ☺ ✿

Nearly all lighting's labeling is highly technical. Indeed, at first glance it might seem like you need an advanced degree to make sense of it. But if you learn a few terms and numbers, you can make better choices about your lighting (plus save some money!). There are four main types of lighting—incandescent, halogen, fluorescent, and LED.

- Least amount of energy used: LED
- Significantly less energy used: fluorescent, including CFLs
- Less energy used: new-technology halogen bulbs
- Most energy used: incandescent (which also produces the most heat from the bulb)

Fluorescent and LED lights use at least 75 percent less energy than incandescents, yet most incandescent and new-technology halogen lights still have the best dimming ability and look. LEDs last the longest (up to twenty years!), produce virtually no heat, have the purest light, and release the least amount of harmful emissions—but are currently the costliest, don't illuminate a whole room, and have limited availability. The good news is that you can expect to see more LED lighting options in the future as the technology evolves. Before you buy your bulbs, think about what you want to light and how you want to light it; this will help you choose your type and look—there are a lot of choices!

- Housecleaning, home office work, and larger-scale craft or hobby work:
    - Daylight-labeled CFL bulb—make sure the packaging says the CFL is dimmable for evening use.
    - Skylight with supplemental CFL, incandescent, or halogen bulb add-in for evening lighting with dimmer switch.
    - Three-way lamp with a daylight-label or a three-way CFL bulb— you can adjust the lamp's lighting depending on the time of day or if any other natural light is available.
    - On the horizon—look for new-generation LED lightbulbs that may radiate light more effectively and light a whole room.

- Bathrooms:
    - CFL with either daylight label or higher lumens on the packaging.
    - Daylight-labeled incandescent or new-generation halogen.

- Lighting that can be spotlight oriented—artwork, decorative lighting, Christmas lights, and craft or hobby work:
  LED light

- Evening light only—for eating dinner and unwinding in the evening:
  Warm-color CFL or new-technology halogen bulb with dimming ability—if you will be doing evening tasks that need truer colors (like painting) or are detailed (like needlework) then you might choose to add an extra side lamp with daylight or cool lighting, or a spotlight-type LED light.

- Outdoor porch light on a motion detector:
  CFL if the light stays on for at least ten minutes; otherwise, choose incandescent, halogen, or LED.

- Outdoor porch lights that are not on a motion detector:
  Warm CFL—no need to spend the extra money on daylight lighting or cooler Kelvin temperatures (see chart below) for this purpose.

>> **Look for lightbulbs with a combination of lower watts and higher lumens—you'll get more light for your buck!**

Here's a handy chart outlining the technical terms you might encounter when choosing your lighting and my easy-to-understand translation.

"WATTS" IT ALL ABOUT	
Technical Terms	**What the Light Will Look Like**
Watts measure how much energy your lightbulb will use.	Choose lights with the *lowest wattage* to save energy and money.
Lumens measure how much light will be produced by your light or lightbulb.	Choose lights with *higher lumens* to get more light and more brightness.

Technical Terms	What the Light Will Look Like
Kelvin (K) measures the color temperature of the light or lightbulb. Kelvin temperature does *not* tell you how hot (to the touch) the bulb will be when lit.	Want a warm-colored light? *Lower Kelvin* numbers mean a *warmer color*. The light will have a more yellowish tint. Example: A 2,700–3,000 K CFL is similar to the warm light of an incandescent bulb. Want a cooler, more daylight-like light? *Higher Kelvin* numbers mean a *cooler color* and come closer to the color of sunlight—daylight lighting. The light will look more white than yellow. Look for 5,000 K or higher for daylight-like light.
Color Rendering Index (CRI) measures how well a light will make the colors in your room look their truest color. A perfect CRI is one hundred. This is the CRI of the sun—and colors look their truest in sunlight. It is more common that daylight-labeled or full-spectrum lighting will list CRI on their packaging.	When you want to simulate sunshine and/or have the truest color rendering, look for a *higher CRI*. Any number above eighty is considered very good.
The UL mark tells you that the lighting product has been tested and is certified to be safe for your use.	Note: The UL mark is not always found on the outside of the package but rather sometimes inside the labeling or box.

Some daylight lighting might have a high K number but does not have a high CRI number. But you want both high K and high CRI if your aim is to find indoor lighting that simulates sunshine.

Don't turn your CFL on and off like a regular lightbulb. Leave it on for at least five to fifteen minutes, otherwise you may shorten its life and brightness. If you rarely use the light and when you do it is only on for a few minutes, then you can stick with a traditional incandescent or a halogen bulb.

get the truth about cfl mercury danger

Like many environmental challenges, lightbulbs are no different in that sometimes you make gains in one area only to encounter problems in another area. It's a sort of trade-off. Take the case of fluorescent lightbulbs—they offer amazing energy efficiency when compared to traditional incandescent lightbulbs, but they also pose a little potential problem called mercury.

Most CFLs are currently made with about 2.5 to 3 milligrams of mercury that is encapsulated into the light—this is equal to about one one-hundredth of the amount of mercury found in a household temperature thermometer. If the light breaks or if it is disposed of in your regular trash bin for collection, mercury vapors can escape into the air, causing a health and environmental hazard. There has been a lot of discussion about this mercury danger, and it is still somewhat controversial.

The National Lighting Bureau (www.nlb.org) says that when a CFL breaks, "most of its mercury adheres to the glass and does not disperse in the air," though you should still follow the Environmental Protection Agency's cleanup guidelines found in this chapter. And, says the Bureau, overall mercury is still being reduced by switching to CFLs: Since much of our electricity is still powered by coal-burning plants, which produce mercury as an atmospheric pollutant, CFLs substantially reduce that electricity production and use when compared with traditional incandescent bulbs.

The EPA advises to recycle CFL bulbs once they burn out by taking them to your city's recycling center—nearly all components of a fluorescent bulb can be recycled in a nonhazardous way, including the mercury. You can save several of these bulbs in a sealed plastic bag and make just one annual trip to the recycling center, disposing of your other hazardous waste like paint and batteries at the same time. As a free service, Home Depot accepts unbroken CFLs for recycling. And, if your fluorescent light accidentally breaks, follow these cleanup guidelines from the EPA.

What to Do if a Fluorescent Lightbulb Breaks *

- Before cleanup: vent the room:
    - Open a window and leave the room for fifteen minutes or more.
    - Shut off the central forced-air heating or air-conditioning system, if you have one.

---

*Courtesy of U.S. Environmental Protection Agency.

- Cleanup steps for hard surfaces:
    - Carefully scoop up glass fragments and powder using stiff paper or cardboard and place the fragments in a glass jar with a metal lid (such as a canning jar) or in a sealed plastic bag.
    - Use sticky tape, such as duct tape, to pick up any remaining small glass fragments and powder.
    - Wipe the area clean with damp paper towels or disposable wet wipes and place them in the glass jar or plastic bag.
    - Do not use a vacuum or broom to clean up the broken bulb on hard surfaces.

- Cleanup steps for carpeting or rugs:
    - Carefully pick up glass fragments and place them in a glass jar with a metal lid (such as a canning jar) or in a sealed plastic bag.
    - Use sticky tape, such as duct tape, to pick up any remaining small glass fragments and powder.
    - Vacuum the area where the bulb was broken.
    - Remove the vacuum bag (or empty and wipe the canister) and put the bag or vacuum debris in a sealed plastic bag.

- Disposal of cleanup materials:
    - Immediately place all cleanup materials outside the building in a trash container or in an outdoor, protected area to be picked up with the next normal trash.
    - Wash your hands after disposing of the jars or plastic bags containing cleanup materials.
    - Check with your local or state government about disposal requirements in your specific area. Some states prohibit such trash disposal and require that broken and unbroken lamps be taken to a local recycling center.

- Future cleaning of carpeting or rugs:
    - Vent the room during and after vacuuming.
    - For at least the next several cleanings, shut off the central forced-air heating or air-conditioning system and open a window prior to vacuuming.

Keep the central heating or air-conditioning system shut off and the window open for at least fifteen minutes after vacuuming is completed.

>> According to Energy Star, CFLs perform best in open fixtures that allow airflow, such as table and floor lamps, wall sconces, pendants, and outdoor fixtures.

FEIT ELECTRIC >> (www.feitelectric.com) Has a variety of lightbulbs, including a low-mercury CFL called ECObulb Plus.

GE >> (www.ge.com) Full range of energy-efficient lighting including the Reveal line of daylight-simulating lightbulbs, now also available as a halogen light which lasts three times longer than incandescent.

LIGHTING SCIENCE GROUP >> (www.lsgc.com) Sells screw-in LED lightbulbs and other quality LED lighting products.

LITEBOOK >> (www.litebook.com) Excellent portable light therapy boxes that use LEDs to simulate the sunshine.

LUMIRAM >> (www.lumiram.com) Daylight and full-spectrum lighting, including CFLs.

OTT-LITE >> (www.ott-lite.com) Daylight lighting lamps, especially good for tasks like reading, sewing, and art.

PHILIPS >> (www.usa.philips.com) Full range of energy-efficient lighting, including daylight lighting and dimmable CFLs; also has a more efficient version of halogen lights, which burn about 20–25 percent cooler than standard incandescents; and has a line of high-quality architectural tricolor LED lights.

SYLVANIA >> (www.sylvania.com) Full range of energy-efficient lighting, including daylight-labeled lighting.

TECHNICAL CONSUMER PRODUCTS >> (www.tcpi.com) Makes a nice warm white CFL lamp that produces light very close to the look of incandescent.

VERILUX >> (www.verilux.com) Daylight and full-spectrum lighting, including CFLs.

Get Rid of Old-Style Halogen Torchiere Lights ☺ $

Old-style halogen torchiere lights can use 300–500 watts of electricity to produce less than fifty lumens of light—that's very expensive, low-level light! Also, these old halogens can get *very* hot and become fire hazards. With all the other lighting options out there, you can probably do much better. First, properly dispose of the old halogen bulb, then look for Energy Star–rated halogen lighting, or look into more efficient options like CFLs.

Install Motion Sensors and Dimmers ☺ ☼ $–$$

If you want to help yourself wind down in the evening, consider installing dimmers on your household lighting. Dimmers are a fabulous thing to have available for evening lighting. As nightfall approaches, you want to be able to relax and turn down the lights—this triggers a natural chemical process in your brain that tells you it's time to unwind and slow down, getting yourself ready for sleep. Dimmers can help you to further reduce your electricity use and extend the life of your bulb. If you install a dimmer switch, be sure that the bulbs you purchase are dimmable—traditionally, incandescent and halogen have offered the best dimming ability and look but CFLs are rapidly improving.

You can also save energy by installing motion sensors (also called sensor light switches). While we often associate motion sensors with outdoor lights, they make sense for your indoor lights as well. Because they'll turn off and on when you need them, you'll spend less time running around turning off lights.

> **LEVITON >>** (www.leviton.com) Full range of lighting switches, including dimmers and motion sensor switches.
>
> **LUTRON >>** (www.lutron.com) High-quality dimmers for energy efficiency and ambiance lighting.

Install Energy Star Lighting Fixtures ☺ $-$$

There's been a lot of talk about changing out your lightbulbs, but you can also improve your lighting energy efficiency by changing the whole fixture. New technology and new engineering have offered advances in light fixtures, and now there are Energy Star–rated ones. Rated fixtures have to keep the light high in lumens (brightness) while keeping the use of watts (electricity) down. Energy Star's Web site (www.energystar.gov) lists rated fixtures.

> **GOOD EARTH LIGHTING >>** (www.goodearthlighting.com) Energy Star–rated lighting fixtures.
>
> **KICHLER LIGHTING >>** (www.kichler.com) Energy Star–rated lighting fixtures.
>
> **MINKA GROUP >>** (www.minka.com) Energy Star–rated lighting fixtures and ceiling fans.
>
> **THOMAS LIGHTING >>** (www.thomaslighting.com) Energy Star–rated lighting fixtures.

Consider Outdoor Solar Lighting ☺ **$$–$$$**

Outdoor solar lighting features small, sky-facing solar panels that gather power from the sun to provide light in the evening. These lamps mainly use LED lights because they require so little power to illuminate. Most outdoor solar lighting is easy to install since the lamps are wireless; however, those that provide backup power or come with remote solar panels do have wiring. And once you purchase your lighting, the power is free—direct from the sun.

tales from a lighting designer

Andris Kasparovics, a graduate of the Purchase College, School of the Arts, Conservatory of Theatre Arts and Film, and a professional lighting designer in San Francisco, has been lighting spaces for over ten years—from homes to commercial buildings to presidential galas. He says that while CFLs have been the leading alternative to incandescent lighting, the technology surrounding LED lighting has also improved greatly in recent years, allowing it to become a very flexible and eco-friendly light source. LED color temperature (Kelvin) on the warm end has improved quite a bit and Kasparovics believes that LED lighting will easily replace incandescent lightbulbs in the next five years.

Here are some of his lighting tips:

- The easiest and most cost-effective route to energy efficiency and environmental protection with lighting is to change all task lights and general room lights to CFLs. Kasparovics had a client who began saving 65 percent on his energy bill immediately after switching all of his lamps to CFLs. Task lights are generally desk lamps, bathroom vanity lighting, and other work-area lighting.
- The wattage of a CFL is much lower than an equivalent lightbulb due to its higher efficiency, so a good ratio would be 3:1 incandescent to CFL wattage. For example, to replace a 75-watt lightbulb you would need a 27-watt CFL.
- In a home environment where you want to relax, choose lower color temperatures, as the warmer tone of the light feels a lot more inviting and provides a much better atmosphere than the colder light from higher color temperature sources.

- CFL lamps are not good for spotlighting or accent lighting, as the light they produce is very soft and nondirectional. LED is better suited to that, as it has the ability to produce a more focused beam with truer color rendering.

- Look for fun ways to light your home, such as with tricolor LEDs that allow you to change the feel or atmosphere of a room just by subtly changing colors. This is a relatively new concept that is opening up a lot of creative possibilities for the homeowner. An example would be to use a light amber or pastel lavender in a wall sconce fixture or in indirect cove lighting, which casts a soft light on the ceiling. Kasparovics has also installed a system for a client that would slowly change the ceiling lighting from a white during the day to a warmer amber color in the evening. Kids' rooms are where he is seeing more color used, such as table lamps or nightlights in cube and sphere shapes that have color-changing LEDs inside.

- Put some of your lights in the least occupied areas, like the garage and basement areas, on motion sensor switches. This way the light only comes on when you enter the room and will turn off when you leave.

LIFESTYLE ACTION

treat household water like gold

what you need to know

If you live in an area that has water shortages, you already know to conserve your household water usage, but even if you live in a rain-soaked location, you also need to conserve. No matter how much water is available, it still takes energy, chemicals, and your money to keep water clean enough to drink and use in your home. Also, all the water that goes down our drains (wastewater) is treated before it is released back into lakes, rivers, oceans, or for nondrinking commercial use; this also takes a lot of energy, money, and public resources.

Since the Clean Water Act of 1972—which has been amended several times since then and will likely continue to be improved to enhance

‚protections—there have been stricter water and wastewater standards put into place to protect humans and the environment; this act has greatly improved the quality of our water and waterways by cutting down on pollution and the dumping of toxic substances. It is important to support clean water legislation so that your water can be protected now, and for future generations.

>> Toilet flushing accounts for nearly a third of all the water you use in your home.

benefits

Clean water protects your health and the health of your family. Certain water conservation methods will lower your water bill, conserve water resources and energy, and send less wastewater to be processed—all of which is good for the environment.

how-to's

Reduce Excess Running Water ☺ $

This sounds like a no-brainer, but shut the water off when it's not needed. Doing this can save water and money. Pay attention to times when you let the water run without using it. For example, when you:

- *Brush your teeth.* You only need the water for wetting the toothbrush and rinsing, not the whole time you brush your teeth.
- *Take a shower.* Whenever possible, keep your showers to under ten minutes.
- *Fill your bath.* Plug the drain from the beginning and let the water warm up as it fills.
- *Shave.* Turn off the water until you need to rinse your razor.

>> Instead of letting your faucet run until you get cold water, cool it down in the refrigerator—you could save one to two gallons of water in the process.

Go Low Flow ☺ $-$$$

You can easily reduce the amount of water your family uses without sacrificing comfort by upgrading your faucets, toilets, and showerheads to low flow versions. Low flow means that the amount of water flowing through the water outlet is reduced. Most household faucet, toilet, and showerhead applications don't need all the extra water flowing through them in order to get the job done.

For showerheads and toilets, you will need to replace the whole fixture or toilet. For faucets, the most inexpensive way you can reduce water flow is to replace the screw-on tip of the faucet with an aerator, which will reduce the water flow by mixing in air with the water. Many new high-efficiency showerheads also use this aerating technology—built directly into the showerhead—and they are engineered so you don't feel as if you're losing out on water comfort or the ability to get a thorough showering. If your showerhead was installed before 1992 it probably has flow rates of 5.5 gallons per minute or higher, so look for a way to replace it with a low-flow version.

For toilets, don't let low flow fool you into thinking your toilet won't flush. The water pressure in the flush isn't changed, only the amount of water used. Most toilets made between 1980 and 1994 use at least 3.5 gallons per flush; today's high-efficiency toilets use less than 1.3 gallons per flush—a big improvement. And there are also dual-flush, high-efficiency toilet options available—another take on low flow. Although Europeans are used to dual-flush toilets, U.S. consumers aren't. Basically, dual-flush toilets have two flushing options: one lever or button mechanism for less waste, and another lever or button mechanism for more waste—just think number one or number two and you get the picture. Dual-flush toilets actually can end up using even less water than low-flow toilets, so they really are super high-efficiency. Look for the WaterSense label on faucets, showerheads, and high-efficiency toilets as a certified indication of their water conservation and quality.

Low-Flow Rates: Rate to Look For

Kitchen faucets: Less than 2.2 gallons per minute
Bathroom faucets: Less than 1.5 gallons per minute

Showerheads: Less than 2.5 gallons per minute
Toilets, high-efficiency: Less than 1.3 gallons per flush

>> Showering with a traditional showerhead uses 5 to 7 gallons
of water per minute, while a low-flow showerhead with only one
head will use no more than 2.5 gallons.

go watersense

An emerging logo that certifies a product's water efficiency is the WaterSense label (www.epa.gov/WaterSense), which is managed by the
EPA. It is a new label that is not yet as widespread as Energy Star, but
will be just as helpful when choosing household products that use water.
Currently it is found on a number of high-efficiency toilets and bathroom
sink faucets. Next, the EPA is planning to add showerheads to the list.
There are no U.S. water-efficiency standards yet for dishwashers, although that is likely to change. Many of the dishwashers sold in the
United States are, however, also sold in Canada, which has its own Energy Star program that rates dishwasher water efficiency; you can do
some online research at the Canadian Energy Star Web site (http
://oee.nrcan.gc.ca/energystar) to find that information.

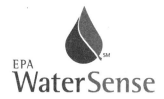

EPA
WaterSense^{SM}

AMERICAN STANDARD >> (www.americanstandard-us.com)
Low-flow and dual-flush toilets and showerheads with high-
efficiency labeling.

(continued)

CRANE PLUMBING >> (www.craneplumbing.com) High-efficiency WaterSense-certified toilets, including dual flush.

DELTA >> (www.deltafaucet.com) Water-efficient showerheads and faucets.

HANSA >> (www.hansaamerica.net) High-efficiency faucets with an additional water-limiting feature to use while you are waiting for the water to heat up.

KOHLER >> (www.kohler.com) High-efficiency toilets (including dual flush) and low-flow faucet fixtures.

MANSFIELD PLUMBING PRODUCTS >> (www.mansfield-plumbing.com) High-efficiency toilets with the WaterSense label, including dual flush.

MOEN >> (www.moen.com) Low-flow, WaterSense-labeled faucets and water-saving showerheads.

PRICE PFISTER >> (www.pricepfister.com) WaterSense-labeled low-flow faucets and aerators that can be installed by consumers.

TOTO USA >> (www.totousa.com) WaterSense-labeled high-efficiency toilets and faucets, including sensor faucets and dual-flush toilets.

WATERPIK >> (www.waterpik.com) Low-flow showerheads.

Fix Indoor Water Leaks ☺ $–$$

Leaks, in either your faucet or your toilet, can add up to a lot of wasted water and money every year. According to the EPA, a leaky faucet can waste more than 3,000 gallons of water per year and a leaky toilet can waste 73,000 gallons of water per year. That's 200 gallons of water per day!

To check if you have a leak, put a bowl under the faucet for a few hours and see if water accumulates. For a leaky toilet, turn the water to the toilet off, open up the tank's lid, and mark the water line with a pencil; if after a couple of hours the water line has descended, then you have a leaky toilet that would have otherwise refilled itself (perhaps over and over) if the water to the toilet had been left on. Many do-it-yourself books can show you how to solve both of these problems on your own. Otherwise, hire a handyman or a plumber to help you either fix the problem or determine if you need a new faucet or toilet.

Reduce Dishwashing Water Usage ☺ $

Whether you wash your dishes by hand or in the dishwasher, you can save water just by changing a few habits. If you are washing by hand several times a day and for a family, generally it will be more energy- and water-efficient to use a dishwasher. But if you are washing a small amount of dishes for just a couple of people, then you can consider washing your dishes by hand with minimal water usage. Otherwise, wait until your dishwasher is full before running it. Because food on plates might become dry and thereby harder for the dishwasher to get off without first running a soak cycle, soak dishes that have food remnants on them in the sink until you're ready to run a load.

If you wash your dishes by hand, fill the sink with water and wash the dishes—then put the soapy-yet-cleaned dishes into a drying rack with a tray on the bottom that can drip excess water into the sink. Use your sink sprayer to rinse the dishes right in the rack all at once. If you don't have a sprayer but do have a dual kitchen sink, you can rinse the washed dishes in the second sink all at once to avoid running the water for a long period of time.

For dishwasher washing, scrape but don't prerinse to save water. The dishwasher soap needs some scum on the dishes in order to work properly—or you can put a pat of butter (to serve as quasi-scum) in the bottom of the dishwasher so that the soap has something to react with. When using your dishwasher, choose the shortest cycle possible, which will reduce water usage. I generally only use the light wash feature on my dishwasher, even if my dishwasher is completely full.

the dish on dishwashers

When you are purchasing a new dishwasher, the Department of Energy recommends you check the EnergyGuide label to see how much energy it uses. Dishwashers fall into one of two categories: compact capacity and standard capacity. Although compact-capacity dishwashers may appear to be more energy efficient on the EnergyGuide label, they hold fewer dishes, which may force you to use it more frequently. In this case, your energy costs could be higher than with a standard-capacity dishwasher. And a built-in heat booster on your dishwasher might cost a little more up front, but it will save you money in the long run because you won't need to turn up your water heater any higher than 120°F. The dishwasher heats on demand.

Wash Your Clothes Using Less Water ☺ ∅-$$$

Laundry is the second-largest use of household water after flushing your toilet. And I can attest to that, with all the laundry that gets done in my house! So, if there's anything you can do to reduce the amount of water you use but still get your clothes spiffy clean, I'm all for it.

Try washing your clothes only when you have enough items to fill the washer—this makes the washing job most worth the effort and water used. Or, if you have a water-level-adjustment feature on your washer, then choose the load size (usually small, medium, or large) which controls how much water you use.

Another option is to buy a front-loading washing machine, which tumbles your clothes to wash them, thereby needing less water than traditional top-loading washers to get the job done. Like front-loading machines, there's also new-technology high-efficiency top-loading washers that use less water, energy, and detergent. Many new front-loading and high-efficiency washers will require you to buy low-sudsing detergent, often represented on the detergent's label by HE for high-efficiency.

Additionally, the new steam-only washers can also freshen and clean lightly soiled clothes without the traditional wear and tear of washing, making your clothes last and look better longer; longevity is helpful to your pocketbook and the environment.

The Department of Energy says that inefficient washing machines can cost three times as much to operate than energy-efficient ones.

When selecting a new machine, look for not only the Energy Star rating but also a feature that allows you to adjust the water temperature and level for different loads. Efficient clothes washers spin-dry your clothes more effectively, too, saving energy when drying as well. Read washing machine labels carefully to assess water-efficiency features:

- Energy Star–rated means it's more water and energy efficient. Energy Star rates clothes washers based on what is called a Modified Energy Factor and Water Factor. An Energy Star–rated washer will save you up to $550 in operating costs over its lifetime compared to a regular machine, and will use 35–50 percent less water. You can find the exact Modified Energy Factor and Water Factor numbers at www.energystar.gov.
- New-technology Features, such as water-saving and energy-saving features, are listed by the manufacturer on the package or its Web site.

BOSCH >> (www.boschappliances.com) Water-saving washers and dishwashers.

KENMORE >> (www.kenmore.com) Washing machines and dishwashers with water-efficiency features and Energy Star ratings.

LG ELECTRONICS >> (www.lge.com) Has a dishwasher and clothes washer with a SenseClean system to adjust water usage according to how dirty the dishes or clothes are. And the company also has an energy-efficient clothes washer with a twenty-minute, steam-only cycle to freshen and reduce wrinkles on clothes, which can reduce trips to the dry cleaner.

MAYTAG >> (www.maytag.com) Water-saving washers and dishwashers.

WHIRLPOOL >> (www.whirlpool.com) Water-saving washers and dishwashers, including an innovative steam-technology washing machine.

CHAPTER THREE

eco-overhaul: great ways to green every room in your house

Electronics and appliances, as well as the homes we live in, all have finite life spans. And when it's time to say goodbye to a computer or a microwave, when you decide to add on or remodel, or if you choose to build an entirely new home, it is important for you to make eco-friendly choices. A vast array of products and services are available that will not only satisfy your need for the latest and greatest technology, but also keep Mother Earth in mind. So when you enter that big-box store or meet up with your contractor, remember to think green.

LIFESTYLE ACTION
plug into smart electronic habits

what you need to know

In my house, we have four televisions. And I'm embarrassed to say it. I wish we didn't have so many, but we've done it entirely for convenience—you know, divide-and-conquer parenting (no one fights over TV programs). We also have three computers, three DVD players, various telephones, stereos, video game players . . . and more. This adds up to lots of power use. And I suspect we're not much different than the average American family in this regard. To prove my point, according to the U.S. Energy Information Administration, by 2015 consumer electronics and small appliances will be responsible for almost 30 percent of all household electricity use.

But even though we're in a wired world, you still need to think green. Primarily you need to consider how much power your electronics are using and reduce that amount. Additionally, as you reduce your power use you will also likely be reducing emissions—invisible gases that pollute the air and the atmosphere, which come out of your electronic products. Over the years there have been a lot of upgrades to electronics to reduce emissions and power consumption. According to the EPA, if all the electronic devices in the United States were replaced by more energy-efficient models, it would save over 25 billion pounds of greenhouse gas emissions each year. This is the equivalent of taking three million cars off the road—a whole lot! This statistic doesn't even take computers and printers into account. Isn't that amazing?

>> **Cut your power usage by limiting the amount of television your children are allowed to watch, and help them find alternate activities that provide for a better-rounded lifestyle.**

benefits

You don't have to sacrifice productivity or fun to save energy and reduce emissions from your electronic devices. Plus, you'll save money!

how-to's

Turn Off What's Not in Use ☺ ∅

Although many of us are trained to turn off lights when we're not in the room, turning off your electronics as well will make a huge difference, especially once you make it a habit. I know that in our home, even though we turn off the TV and all the lights at night, we used to leave the computers on. When we began turning them off each night, we immediately saved about twenty to thirty dollars each month on our electricity bill. Another idea: If you find out that your family is watching the same television program on two TVs in the same house (our family has been guilty of this!), turn off one television set and watch the same program together on one TV. When you won't be at your desk for a while, you can also turn off the computer monitor to save energy.

>> Don't rely on your computer's screensaver for energy savings. Contrary to what many people think, the screensaver is only saving your screen, *not* energy. So skip the screensaver and program your computer to automatically switch to sleep mode instead.

Take Advantage of Power-Saver Modes ☺ ∅

Many newer electronic devices, including many Energy Star–rated ones, are equipped with power-saver modes. Sometimes these are called "sleep" or "standby" mode. Take advantage of them. When in this mode, the device will actually automatically power down to minimal power use when you step away; this results in much less energy wasted, which will save you money, too. Power-saver mode may also mean that you can still use the device but with less features. For example, some TVs in power-saver mode may sacrifice some picture quality and brightness to cut power usage and save you money; but if your room is dimly lit while you watch, you might not even notice the difference.

>> If you own an LCD television, read your owner's manual to find out how to reduce the intensity of your backlight. You'll save power by doing this.

XBOX >> (www.xbox.com) Game console with a sleep mode to conserve energy during long downloads (which can take several hours) and a timer that can be set to restrict the amount of time spent playing games.

Completely Unplug Your Device ☺ ∅

This is different than just hitting the off switch. You can save a few more watts of power (sometimes a lot more, depending on the product) by completely unplugging the device from the outlet on the wall, which cuts off phantom power. Phantom power is electricity usage that can happen when your electronic device has the switch turned off but is not unplugged. In other words, "off" doesn't really mean "off." Many of today's electronics still use power in the off mode (which should really be called "hibernation mode") so that when you turn them on, they will wake up quickly or respond to a remote control in an instant. You might be surprised to learn that 40 percent of the energy used by home electronics is consumed when these products are in hibernation mode. So, to save yourself energy (and money!), unplug each device from the wall when you're done using it, or attach several devices (such as TVs, DVD players, and stereos) to one power strip so that you can unplug several products at once with one pull—my favorite way.

But note that completely unplugging some electronics can have side effects. For example, if I completely unplug my computer and its peripherals, I then have to reset my Internet router when I turn it on again (not a fun task). Also, some devices have settings that might be lost if completely unplugged. I, for one, hate breaking out the manual just to reset the clock. A good rule of thumb is that whatever happened during your last power outage is what will happen when you unplug.

>> The Alliance to Save Energy says that Americans are spending more money to power audio and DVD electronics *when they're off* compared to when they're on. It's all that sneaky phantom power at work.

Replace Your Electronics with Energy-Efficient Models ☺ ✿ $-$$$$

If you have the budget to start upgrading, you can start buying energy-efficient electronics to cut down your power needs for those devices by as much as 50 percent—without sacrificing fun or productivity. Look for the Energy Star label when you shop for energy-efficient electronics. It should be obviously placed right on the product's packaging.

Unfortunately, not all types of electronics have an Energy Star–rated option. Do your online and in-store research to determine how much energy a product will save you. This means noting how many watts it uses, estimated annual energy cost, power-saver mode options, and how much energy is used in phantom or standby mode. But be practical. Don't run out and buy an energy-saving device unless there's a big difference between what you already have and the newest product on the market. There's no reason to dump old products into your landfill or city's recycling program if you can help it. Sometimes simply powering an electronics device down when you're not using it can save as much or more energy than using the newest power-saving device.

APPLE >> (www.apple.com) Computer products and electronics with Energy Star ratings, and power consumption management features. Company follows more responsible manufacturing practices.

DELL >> (www.dell.com) Comprehensive environmental initiatives for its electronics and computers, such as phasing out toxic substances from their products, adding in energy-efficiency features, computers made from recycled parts, and free recycling of any Dell, anytime.

EPSON >> (www.epson.com) Sells Energy Star–rated electronics. The company has an extensive recycling program; a goal of zero waste in its manufacturing, which also saves resources; programs to reduce packaging; and a control initiative to eliminate harmful substances and replace them with safer alternatives.

HEWLETT-PACKARD >> (www.hp.com) Computers and other office equipment with eco-friendly and energy-saving features like Energy Star ratings, mercury-free displays, and power-saving options. Recycled plastics are also used in their printers.

LENOVO >> (www.lenovo.com) Energy Star–rated computer products with energy-efficient and eco-friendly features like lower power consumption and mercury-free LED displays. Their ThinkPad laptops are made with plastics recycled from water bottles. Products are made to be recycled at the end of their life.

LG ELECTRONICS >> (www.lge.com) Has eco-designed appliances and electronics that are focused on efficiency, energy reduction, less hazardous materials in manufacturing, and more recyclability.

NEC DISPLAY >> (www.necdisplay.com) Energy Star–rated display screens and monitors; company has a recycling program.

PANASONIC >> (www.panasonic.com) Focuses on many environmental initiatives, including Energy Star certification, refurbishment of PC notebooks, and electronics recycling.

PHILIPS >> (www.usa.philips.com) Philips electronics offer built-in energy savings as well as additional power-saver functions such as rechargeable batteries for some of its smaller products. They have won awards for their eco-initiatives.

PIONEER >> (www.pioneerelectronics.com) Energy Star–certified electronic products with energy-save mode.

SAMSUNG >> (www.samsung.com) Extensive green management initiatives to reduce packaging, add power-saving features, and introduce a reusable notebook PC.

SONY ELECTRONICS >> (www.sony.com) Dedicated to environmentally conscious new electronics such as eco-friendly notebook computers and low-power-use organic OLED televisions. OLED stands for organic light-emitting diode and is used primarily for screens like television or computer screens; OLED offers significantly less power consumption than traditional liquid crystal displays (LCDs) because they do not require a backlight. However, OLED screens currently do not last as long as a nonorganic LCD or LED screen.

TOSHIBA >> (www.toshiba.com) Showing considerable commitment to the environment and public health by phasing out PVC and BFRs (see page 165) from *all* of its products, and offers to take back and recycle its computers and televisions.

Use the Microwave to Save Power ☺ ☼

You can save energy by using the microwave to reheat or cook small portions of food. One of my favorite ways to use the microwave is for baked potatoes—I keep my oven off for the one to two hours it would have taken to bake them, saving 50 percent of the energy that I would have used in oven cooking (not to mention the time saved). And my baked potatoes still taste great. Also, microwave use does not heat up the kitchen so much as an oven, which could save you money on your air-conditioning bills. If you are cooking a larger meal, it will likely be more efficient to use the stove and oven.

Use a Programmable Thermostat as an Energy-Saving Tool ☺ ☼ $$

Growing up, we managed the heating and cooling manually with the thermostat on the wall. But today we have a better way—programmable thermostats for your heating and cooling system. A programmable thermostat can more readily and accurately manage desired temperatures, especially for different times of day. You can set it to maintain more comfortable temperatures when you're home, and be colder (in the winter) or warmer (in the summer) when you're away at work. Most utility companies recommend ideal temperature settings of seventy-eight degrees for the summer and sixty-eight degrees or lower during the winter. Look for the Energy Star logo when making this purchase—Energy Star thermostats will contain no mercury (a toxic health risk) and when used properly, can save you about $150 a year on your heating and cooling costs when compared with a manual thermostat.

Be Smart About Space Heating ☺ ☼

Don't use a space heater to heat up large rooms or the whole residence, because generally they aren't energy efficient for these big jobs. Instead, use them to warm small spaces. Radiant portable heaters are a great choice because they don't circulate air, but rather radiate heat to warm people and objects near the unit; radiant heaters are also more energy efficient than traditional forced-air heaters (the fan-type heaters) and pose less fire risks than traditional forced-air heaters.

INDUS-TOOL >> (www.indus-tool.com) Energy-efficient radiant portable heaters.

>> Want to cut down on your heating bill? How about this tried-and-true approach—wear a sweater! Take advantage of capturing your own body heat for warmth instead of using more electricity or gas.

Clean or Replace Your Central Air Filter Regularly ☺ ∅

It isn't difficult to understand that if you have a dirty air filter it will be more difficult for air to flow through it. I put a little note on the first day of every month to check my air filter and see if it needs to be replaced. Although a once-a-month filter check is a good rule of thumb, in some climates families don't use the central air system every month, so your filter will not be dirty. Some air filters are washable and only need to be wiped or sprayed clean—this is ideal because reuse of any product is better for the environment and your pocketbook. Other filters, however, need to be tossed in the trash and completely replaced.

Get Regular Maintenance on Your Cooling (and Heating) System ☺ $$

Just as your car needs regular maintenance to remain in good working order, so too do your heating and cooling units. Although you can easily change or wash air filters, it is best to hire a contractor for an annual checkup. Professional maintenance keeps your system(s) working at top performance levels to give you the biggest bang for your buck. According to Energy Star, you should expect the following from your contractor when your system is checked:

- Thermostat settings and functionality are checked.
- All electrical connections are checked.
- All moving parts are lubricated as necessary to prevent friction and early wear.

- Drains are checked and unplugged as necessary.
- System cycles are run to make sure the controls work properly.
- Any coils are cleaned.
- Refrigerant levels are checked.
- Gas connections and burners are examined for any possible problems.
- Airflow is checked.

Buy Green Power ✚

Buying your power from more renewable energy sources (such as wind, solar, or geothermal) is the wave of the future and most likely coming to a state near you. When you buy greener power, you are helping to clean the air and water in your surrounding region. You are also supporting technologies that will last and improve the sustainability of your community. Unfortunately, at the present time most green power will cost you a bit more than conventional power by charging you a premium per kilowatt-hour (kWh)—but it often turns out to be two to ten dollars more per month for the average resident, not hundreds of dollars. Your utility company will likely have information online that explains the program(s) offered, how to sign up, and what extra costs you may expect.

> **THE GREEN POWER NETWORK >>** (www.eere.energy.gov/greenpower) This is a useful site from the Department of Energy that helps you find green power options where you live.

LIFESTYLE ACTION

purchase energy-saving appliances

what you need to know

By choosing more energy-efficient appliances, you can save at least a third if not more on the energy you would have spent keeping an antiquated appliance running. Additionally, energy-saving appliances produce less greenhouse gases, so you're making a positive impact on the earth and are investing in the health of your family. If you have to choose which of your old appliances to get rid of and replace first, consider your refrigerator. The fridge is always on, so it will reap the most energy savings right away.

to change or not to change

If your major appliance is more than twelve to fifteen years old, it is highly likely that there have been sufficient technological gains in energy efficiency for that type of appliance, and perhaps eco-friendly features and manufacturing, to warrant a replacement. Just make sure you recycle or donate your old appliance.

benefits

You will save at least a third on your energy costs by replacing your appliances with more energy-efficient models, and this will also help you to protect the environment.

how-to's

Look for the Energy Star Label ☺ ∅

The Energy Star label is the most reliable way for you to determine if an appliance or household electronic item will use energy more efficiently. It is found on products in more than fifty categories for your home or office (more than 40,000 individual products and 2,000 manufacturers), including office equipment, home electronics, heating and cooling units, major appliances like washers and refrigerators, water heaters, lighting fixtures, and windows. The label was created in 1992 to help you save money and to protect the environment by reducing greenhouse gas emissions.

When you purchase a household product that has earned the Energy Star label, it guarantees that you will be able to operate that product using less energy (10–90 percent, depending on the product and its other features) than if you had purchased a standard product. An Energy Star rating on a washer means it will use less water than conventional models.

You should also look into any available federal or state tax credits given for purchasing an Energy Star product; your city and your utility company may also offer rebates or incentives. That's money in your pocket just for looking for an Energy Star label. Here is a sample of the label:

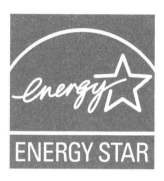

>> The Energy Star label does not rate whether or not there are less hazardous materials being used in a product.

>> According to the Department of Energy, the cost of running an Energy Star refrigerator is less than the cost of running a regular 75-watt lightbulb.

BOSCH >> (www.boschappliances.com) Company provides high-quality appliances and has a long-term commitment to rating all of its appliances with the Energy Star certification—for energy-efficient cooking, laundry, and dishwashing.

ELECTROLUX >> (www.electrolux.com) Full line of Energy Star-rated appliances, including ovens, ranges, dishwashers, and refrigerators.

GE >> (www.ge.com) Many energy-efficient and Energy Star appliances.

KENMORE >> (www.kenmore.com) Many energy-efficient, high-quality household appliances with interesting technological advances.

LG ELECTRONICS >> (www.lge.com) Has eco-designed appliances and electronics that are focused on efficiency, energy reduction, less hazardous materials in manufacturing, and more recyclability.

MAYTAG >> (www.maytag.com) High-efficiency and Energy Star–rated household laundry and kitchen appliances.

WHIRLPOOL >> (www.whirlpool.com) Energy Star–rated appliances for the kitchen, laundry, and whole home.

Comparison Shop with the EnergyGuide Label ☺ ∅
When you are researching new appliances, look for the EnergyGuide label, which offers information about a product's projected energy usage. Based on U.S. Government tests, the label:

- Estimates your energy consumption on a scale that shows energy use in a range with other similar models—the lower this number, the better; this means the appliance will cost less to run.
- Gives you an estimated dollar figure for the product's annual operating cost. This makes shopping a lot easier if you simply compare the EnergyGuide labels of various products.

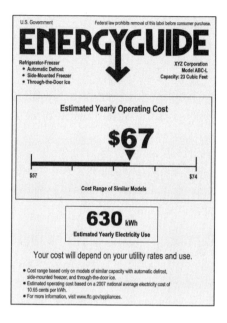

consortium-minded

Although Energy Star and the EnergyGuide label are the most consumer-friendly avenues to information about a product's energy efficiency, the Consortium for Energy Efficiency (www.cee1.org) also offers useful information. This organization works mostly with public utilities, environmental groups, research organizations, and state energy offices alongside partnerships with manufacturers, retailers, and other government agencies to promote the manufacture and purchase of energy-efficient products.

Although the information provided by the Consortium for Energy Efficiency is more technical and can test your ability to understand engineering language, there are databases on the Web site that categorize household products into tiers with the highest tiers being the most efficient. I have found this information really helpful for comparing products; in some cases only the higher-tiered products qualify for rebates.

Consider Small Appliances ☺ $–$$$

Although it's more efficient to buy one larger refrigerator than two smaller ones, you might consider investing in some small appliances for just the right jobs to save energy. The best examples of small appliances that can save energy are microwaves and toaster ovens.

Save By Convection ☺ ✿ $$$-$$$$

If you are in the market for a new oven, take a look at convection ovens. They are usually more energy efficient because the heated air is circulated within the oven while cooking, which means that the temperature is maintained more readily and your food cooks faster. A convection oven can save about 20 percent of energy compared with a conventional oven. However, if you buy a portable version, make sure it is thoroughly insulated to maintain the energy efficiency.

Look into Getting a Tankless Water Heater ☺ $$$-$$$$

A great example of how new appliance technology can save you money and help the environment is a tankless water heater. Traditional water heaters have a tank that constantly uses energy to keep the water at a desired temperature (usually 120°F). Since we rarely turn off the water heater when we leave home, such as during the workday or when we go on vacation, that water is being heated for no reason. With a tankless water heater, the water is heated on an as-needed basis; it travels quickly through a heating element and is tuned to the desired temperature.

The newest tankless water heaters can save you about 70 percent on fuel if you are replacing an old water heater, and they are compact. Plus, many versions qualify for rebates from your public utility or government. When making your selection, you need to know:

- What is the water heater's purpose? Will it heat water entering the whole house, or just portions of a home, like one bathroom or a washing machine, outdoor sink, or pool?
- How will the water heater be powered? By electric or gas power? What kind of voltage or amperage will you need— dedicated circuit breaker or other venting requirements?
- What is the incoming water temperature? What is the desired heated temperature? Knowing this will help you determine if the tankless system will have enough power to heat the water to the desired degree.

Even if you don't replace your traditional water heater with a tankless system, you can change the temperature setting on the water heater to save energy and money. Many water heaters come preset with a desired temperature of 140°F. But most homes only need 120°F, as long as your dishwasher has a heat booster to bring up the temperature.

RHEEM >> (www.smarterhotwater.com) Tankless water heaters with low-emissions features.

LIFESTYLE ACTION

build and remodel green

what you need to know

Whether you build your home from the ground up or remodel, there is a major opportunity to improve the health and safety of your everyday life and reduce the impact that your living space will have on your environment. Building green may cost you slightly more up front, but you are guaranteed savings once you move in. And as with any building or remodeling, you can make choices: reducing air pollution in your home through lower emissions, reducing energy and water usage, decreasing the toxicity of items installed in your home, and using more eco-friendly, responsible, and renewable materials.

THE GREEN HOUSE >> (www.nbm.org) Look under 2007 exhibitions for the Green House at this Web site of the National Building Museum. There are tons of ideas and product listings from this sustainable living and architecture exhibit.

benefits

Your health and safety can be significantly improved, plus it will help the environment. Don't forget about the cost savings, both immediate and for the long haul.

how-to's

Look into LEED Certification ✚ ✿ ☺

The U.S. Green Building Council (www.usgbc.org) administrates a Leadership in Energy and Environmental Design (LEED), a third-party certification of new construction and remodeling materials and projects that have less impact on the environment (less emissions, more responsible, renewable, and nontoxic materials being put into the building); are healthier for those who work and/or live in the building (better air quality, lower risk for mold and mildew); and save money (more energy and water efficiency). Whole homes can be LEED certified, and you can remodel according to LEED guidelines. And sometimes there are discounts and rebates offered. Additional information can be found at www.greenhomeguide.org. By looking for LEED-certified materials, you can save time in determining what are possible eco-friendly, more healthy materials for your construction or remodel project.

tools of the trade

Besides LEED certification, you can also look for Energy Star–certified and EnergyGuide-labeled products (as mentioned earlier in this chapter) for energy savings; the WaterSense certification discussed in chapter 2 for water conservation; the Green Seal label (see chapter 4) for low-VOC paints and coatings; the NRFC rating (see chapter 1) for more energy-efficient doors, windows, and skylights; and forest management certifications like the Forest Stewardship Council logo (as noted in chapter 8) for any wood products.

Two other seals that can assist you in saving time in finding more eco-friendly and safe building and remodeling materials and products are:

- Cradle to Cradle (www.c2ccertified.com): This is a certification of many remodeling and building products. The focus is on promoting reusability and recyclability so products don't end up in landfills at the end of their use.
- GREENGUARD (www.greenguard.org): This is a certification for indoor products that have low emissions. The Web site has a searchable database, including a search for flooring, doors, insulation, paints, and wall finishes.

replacing cabinets? do it the green way

If you are going to replace your kitchen or bath cabinets, or even if you are building from the ground up, look for more environmentally responsible and healthier ways to do it.

Try to find another home for your used cabinetry by posting its availability on a recycling Web site like Freecycle (www.freecycle.org) or with a free classified ad on Craigslist (www.craigslist.org); otherwise, contact your city's recycling center for their recommendation and possible pickup.

When it comes to buying new cabinetry, you can use the Environmental Stewardship Program seal as a guide (www.greencabinet source.org). It is a certification by the Kitchen Cabinet Manufacturers Association that shows a manufacturer has created cabinetry meeting environmental requirements in air quality, resources used, and manufacturing.

> **IKEA >>** (www.ikea.com) Environmentally conscious vendor of home furnishing products.
>
> **HANSEN LIVING >>** (www.hansenliving.com) Makes eco-friendly long-lasting kitchens and bathrooms out of wood from responsibly managed forests.

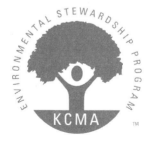

Reduce Your VOCs ✚

With any remodel or building you do, you want to take special care to improve indoor air quality. You help to achieve this by looking for no- or low-VOC products and materials, such as carpets, flooring, or paint. VOCs are volatile organic compounds that give off emissions that pollute the air you breathe and are harmful for the environment. You can look into carpets made of renewable or more eco-friendly fibers with no or low VOCs. Or consider not putting in carpets at all, which is the most air quality–friendly thing you can do; instead, consider such options as sealed concrete, bamboo (that is made with formaldehyde-free glues), or tile flooring. Avoid any vinyl flooring as that is usually made with PVC plastic, which gives off harmful emissions. Also, paint with no- or low-VOC paints.

>> Choose carpet installers that are committed to getting your old carpet recycled.

AFM SAFECOAT >> (www.afmsafecoat.com) Zero-VOC paints and sealers.

BENJAMIN MOORE & CO. >> (www.benjaminmoore.com) Has an Eco Spec line of paints that is lower-odor and low-VOC.

AMERICAN CLAY >> (www.americanclay.com) LEED-certified wall finishing that has zero VOCs, is antimicrobial, and is made of recycled content.

FLOR >> (www.florisgreen.com) Sells very interesting and DIY-friendly carpet tiles that are low in VOCs and are formaldehyde-free. The company also helps its customers recycle old carpets—FLOR arranges for the carpet to be picked up, returned, and recycled at no cost to you.

MERIDA MERIDIAN >> (www.meridameridian.com) Natural fiber woven floor coverings, which include the use of sisal, seagrass, jute, paper, and wool.

MILLIKEN CARPET >> (www.millikencarpet.com) Has green choices for flooring and wall coverings. The company has a recycling program for its customers' carpet tile, saving it from being dumped into landfills. More information is available at www .sustainablecarpet.com.

MYTHIC >> (www.mythicpaint.com) Sells paint that is noncarcinogenic, with zero VOCs and zero toxins.

OLYMPIC >> (www.olympic.com) Has a line of premium interior paints with zero VOCs and the Green Seal of approval.

SHERWIN-WILLIAMS >> (www.sherwin-williams.com) Has a Duration Home line of paints with lower VOCs and a Harmony paint line with fewer solvents and zero VOCs.

TREX >> (www.trex.com) Makes decking, railing, fencing, and trim with reclaimed or recycled safe plastic and wood fibers.

the magic of bamboo

Bamboo is showing up in products everywhere—flooring, countertops, household products, clothing, and much more. It is a remarkable plant in that it is completely sustainable and quick growing, requires no pesticides or fertilizers, and is considered antimicrobial. For example, a typical hardwood tree like oak or teak will take about forty to fifty years to mature. However, commercial timber bamboo is a superhero plant—it grows to its full height in two years, arrives at full maturity in four years, and can then be harvested as usable wood. Additionally, the whole plant doesn't need to be cut down to harvest—only the ripe stems are cut, while others stems continue growing. This makes for a nearly endless cycle of wood for which bamboo forests are not depleted.

It is unlikely that the bamboo you are buying would be coming from forests where pandas live, as timber-use bamboo is often a different type of bamboo than what is eaten by pandas. But it is always good to do some research on this subject before you buy, including whether or not the manufacturer claims it to be farmed organically. Currently, there is no organic label given to bamboo.

Reduce Your Land Footprint ☺

When you have the opportunity to purchase a property and build, consider leaving as much of the land as possible to native habitat. In some cases, this may mean that you have the opportunity to restore native habitat, plant native trees, and give back to the land. With the environment and money savings in mind, your living space or commercial building should only use as much space as is needed for the actual construction. Avoid putting concrete or asphalt over areas that are not needed for driving or storage.

CHAPTER FOUR

clean green: getting down and dirty, the eco-friendly way

Your home is the epicenter of your life. Inside its walls, you and your family cook, eat, play . . . the list is endless. Tons of everyday events—mealtime, for instance—produce waste, necessitate a cleanup, or both. Because disposing of waste and cleaning up our homes are things we do all the time, it's crucial to exert a green effort when we undertake these tasks. And because cooking and cleaning are primo chore categories, the tips in this chapter offer great ways to get your whole family involved in a fantastic, eco-friendly effort.

LIFESTYLE ACTION

dispose with the least amount of harm

what you need to know

Your trash is a big deal—literally. Each of us contributes a lot to trashing up our planet. According to the EPA, in 2006 U.S. residents, businesses, and institutions produced more than 251 million tons of municipal solid waste (MSW), which is approximately 4.6 pounds of waste per person per day. Only 82 million tons of this waste was recycled, which is about a third of the overall waste from that year. Nevertheless, this recycling rate has tremendously increased from almost thirty years ago; in 1980 the rate was just 10 percent and the rest of the waste was either burned or sent to landfills. In fact, although garbage-burning facilities can reduce the amount of waste going to landfills by up to 90 percent in volume and 75 percent in weight, they produce harmful emissions that have serious environmental consequences. The bottom line is we must do a better job of reducing our waste and recycling. The amazing fact is that we really wouldn't be throwing much away—off to be buried in our landfills forever—if we took the time to sort our trash and get nearly all of it recycled or reused. According to the EPA, recycling stops the emission of many greenhouse gases, prevents water from being polluted, saves energy, provides raw materials to industries that can repackage the recycled products into new materials to be reused, creates jobs, stimulates the development of greener technologies, conserves resources for our children's future, and reduces the need for new landfills and garbage-burning facilities. Many cities and states have put a lot of emphasis on recycling, set goals, and met them. California reached 54 percent in waste diversion in 2006, meeting a state-imposed mandate. This means 54 percent of what would otherwise be trash was instead either reused, recycled, or composted (an organic form of recycling). California's rate is particularly high in comparison to most other states, but your state has a waste management board or division that can give you figures and will likely have its own goals and initiatives.

Another area of concern is hazardous household waste—things like paints, cleaners, oils, batteries, pesticides, fertilizers, and portions of electronics and lightbulbs. These items are dangerous if put in the general waste collection and must be given special attention.

In all, since human beings are the source of all this trash, it's up to us to do something about it.

>> Although garbage-burning facilities can reduce the amount of waste going to landfills by up to 90 percent in volume and 75 percent in weight, they produce harmful emissions that have serious environmental consequences.

benefits

By doing your part to reduce what goes to landfills and focusing on reusing and recycling, you can improve your family's air quality, environment, health, and future.

no easy disappearing act

Take a look at how long it takes your trash to decompose in a landfill. Hopefully this might make you and your family more motivated to reduce your use of certain items and to recycle. (Adapted from information available from the U.S. Department of Energy.)

Banana peel:	3–4 weeks
Paper box:	1–2 months
Cotton sock:	5–6 months
Wood:	10–20 years
Leather belt:	40–50 years
Aluminum can:	200–500 years
Disposable diaper:	500–600 years
Styrofoam cup:	1 million years or more
Plastic bottle:	1 million years or more
Glass bottle:	1 million years or more

You can keep your stuff out of landfills through a resource called The Freecycle Network (www.freecycle.org). It is a volunteer organization that helps you post things you want to give away for free (or you can search for particular items as well), such as couches, beds, pianos, tables, chairs, clothes, and building supplies. Think of it as an enormous online garage sale, except everything is free!

Eighty-two million tons of this waste was recycled, which is about a third of the overall waste from that year. This recycling rate has tremendously increased from almost thirty years ago, when in 1980 the rate was just 10 percent and the rest of the waste was either burned or sent to landfills.

how-to's

Get Serious About Trash Sorting and Rerouting ✚ ∅

One of the best, free green things you can do is to sort your trash—and be serious about it. So many of us simply dump everything into the catchall garbage bin or Dumpster. But in order for your environment and health to be protected for now and the future, you need to stop that practice. Here are the main categories to sort your trash:

- Recyclable
- Compostable
- Hazardous (anything labeled flammable, corrosive, an irritant, toxic, or poisonous)
- Donatable
- Green (like garden clippings—you can use some or all of your green in your compost)
- Anything else

Many municipalities provide homes and apartment complexes with three bins: general, recycling, and green waste. And some cities will also provide you with a free outdoor composter. Diligently sort your trash and use those bins. If you live in an apartment-type setting, see if your facility offers separate recycling bins. No matter what your living arrangement is, you will need to secure hazardous waste on your property until you can take it to your municipality's recycling or waste center (as designated by your local waste department) or until your municipality has special collection opportunities (which in many cities are ongoing and are often advertised in your utility bill). You can also make yourself aware of nonprofit organizations or businesses that have recycling programs; some programs are free, others charge a nominal fee, and others give cash for returning bottles.

Although most people have garbage cans throughout their home for general waste, be sure to add at least one inside recycling bin. Add one in your kitchen (no garbage bag needed), your home office area, and your bathroom. This will help ease the collection of recyclable materials for deposit in your recycling bin.

stop the junk

Although you can continue to recycle your junk mail, a better strategy is to put a stop to it coming in the first place. You won't be able to completely get to zero, but you can stem the flow. Some services have cropped up to help you reduce your junk mail—they'll charge you, but it could save you some time. Here are some free tools to reduce junk mail:

- Write a letter or go online to opt out of unsolicited sales pitches—contact your bank, your credit cards, your school (if university or college), your catalogs, and your grocery store and drug store discount card programs.

- Call 1-888-5-OPTOUT to contact all three credit reporting agencies (TransUnion, Experian, and Equifax) to opt out of receiving their mail offers.
- The Center for a New American Dream (www.newdream.org) Educational and junk-mail reducing links.
- Direct Marketing Association (www.dmaconsumers.org) You can contact this organization to remove yourself from mailing lists and prescreened credit offer lists.
- Contact those to whom you pay your bills and ask for paperless billing. Your bills aren't junk, but they could be added waste if you don't mind paperless billing (online).

Services to reduce junk mail:

- Green Dimes (www.greendimes.com)
- 41 Pounds (www.41pounds.org)

trashy truth

Here is a guide that can help you see what to do with your waste in the most environmentally friendly way. Consult your local municipality and state requirements to familiarize yourself with their specific guidelines, as this is only a general guide.

- Rinse all containers that go into recycling bins and flatten if possible.
- Remove all caps from containers that go into recycling bins—it will be doing your recycling facility a favor.
- It helps to remove staples from paper, books, and cardboard— but not all recycling facilities require you to.
- Your city's recycling center should have clearly marked bins for you to place your items in. If you have questions, ask. Some recycling programs (such as for cell phones and eyeglasses) might be located indoors in an administrative area.

- Look for collection days that bring the recycling center curbside for your hazardous or nonbin items—this can save you time.
- Look for special community programs that collect recyclable and reusable items like cell phones, glasses, shoes, and clothing
- You can also call 1-800-CLEANUP for localized information on recycling and hazardous waste disposal.

Type of Waste	Where to Dispose of It
*Aerosol cans that contain *nonhazardous* items like whipped cream and cooking oil	• Recycling bin
*Aerosol cans that contain *hazardous* substances like spray paint and bug spray	• City hazardous waste collection
Aluminum cans	• Recycling bin
Aluminum scrap such as chairs and screens	• Recycling center
Aluminum foil	• Recycling bin
Appliances	• Retailer (when you buy a new appliance, many retailers will take your old appliance and get it to a recycling or reburbishing facility) • Recycling center (you can often call for a special pickup of these items because they are so heavy) • Appliances recycler like JACO Environmental (www.jacoinc.net)
Automobile	• Resell • Retailer (do a trade-in) • Donate (many charity organizations will take used cars and then resell them or sell them to auto recyclers)
*Batteries (non-rechargeable)	• City hazardous waste collection
*Batteries (rechargeable)	• Recycling center • Rechargeable Battery Recycling Corporation (www.rbrc.org)
Books	• Donate (to the local library) • Recycling bin (paperback) • Recycling center (hardback)

Asterisked items are considered hazardous waste

(continued)

Type of Waste	Where to Dispose of It
Bottles (plastic and glass)	• Recycling bin
Boxes (cardboard, detergent, and other household items like cereal boxes)	• Recycling bin
Cans (food and drink)	• Recycling bin
*Car batteries	• Recycling center
*Car waste (oil, antifreeze, filters, and fluids other than water)	• Recycling center
Cardboard (including boxes)	• Recycling bin
Cartons (such as juice and milk cartons)	• Recycling bin
Catalogs	• Recycling bin
CDs	• First, see if you can donate them to a library, school, or another organization that will use them • Recycling center
Cell phones	• Recycling center • Collective Good, an organization that collects and recycles mobile phones (www.collectivegood.com) • Recellular recycles phones (www.recellular.com) • Virgin Mobile recycling service (www.virginmobileusarecycle.com)
Christmas trees	• Recycling center (for real trees) • Special curbside recycling collection (for real trees) • Donate (for artificial trees) • City hazardous waste collection (for artificial trees)
*Cleaners (including car wax)	• City hazardous waste collection
Clothing	• Donate (through charitable organizations) • Reuse (cut up and use as cleaning rags) • Recycling center (for fiber reprocessing)

Asterisked items are considered hazardous waste

Type of Waste	Where to Dispose of It
*Computers	• Recycling center • Donate: Share the Technology is a portal organization that can help you find a place to donate your computer or recycle it (http://sharetechnology.org)
*Disinfectants	• City hazardous waste collection
Dry cleaning items	• Bags (either recycling bin, recycling center, or a special recycling bin for plastic bags at your local grocery store—consult your local municipality) • Hanger (your dry cleaner) • Foam on hanger (your dry cleaner) • Pins (your dry cleaner) • Metal tacks (recycling center) • Cardboard (recycling bin)
DVDs	• Tissue paper (recycling bin) • First, see if you can donate to a library, school, or another organization that will use them • Recycling center
*Electronics	• Recycling center (anything electronic should be accepted) • City hazardous waste collection (depends on if recycling center has an electronics recycling program or not) • Staples stores (nominal fee for recycling electronics brought directly into the store—used computers, monitors, laptops, desktop printers, faxes, and all-in-ones are accepted)
Envelopes	• Recycling bin
Eyeglasses	• Recycling center
File folders	• Recycling bin
*Fire extinguisher	• City hazardous waste collection
*Fluorescent lights	• Recycling center

Asterisked items are considered hazardous waste   (continued)

Type of Waste	Where to Dispose of It
Food trays (such as ones from microwavable meals)	• Recycling bin
Food	• Compost all food waste except bones, meat, and oils/fats
*Fuel (gas, propane, and other fuels)	• City hazardous waste collection
Furniture (tables, chairs, sofas)	• Donate (if repairable or reusable) • Trash bin
Glass	• Recycling bin
Grease (from the kitchen, like meat grease, butter, shortening, and cooking oil)	• Pour into a used can to solidify, then throw it into the trash bin • Do *not* pour down the drain
Hair (from brushes or drains)	• Compost
Hearing aids	• Recycling center
*Helium tanks	• City hazardous waste collection
Junk mail	• Recycling bin (tear up beforehand if your personal information is on it)
Lawn mowers, blowers, and weed eaters	• Recycling center
*Lighter fluid	• City hazardous waste collection
Lint	• Compost
Magazines	• Recycling bin
Mail (paper, cardboard)	• Recycling bin (tear up beforehand if your personal information is on it)
Mattresses	• Donate (some organizations that receive mattresses are able to reuse them; others will disassemble the mattresses to sort and sell the resulting recyclable materials) • Retailer (when you buy a new mattress, many retailers will take your old mattress and get it to a recycling facility)

Asterisked items are considered hazardous waste

Type of Waste	Where to Dispose of It
*Medications	• City hazardous waste collection (do not flush down the toilet or pour down the drain because they can contaminate waterways, oceans, and our drinking water)
*Mothballs	• City hazardous waste collection
*Nail polish remover (such as acetone)	• City hazardous waste collection
Newspaper	• Recycling bin
Newspaper plastic cover	• Either recycling bin (if allowed), recycling center, or a special recycling bin at your local grocery store (consult your local municipality)
*Oily rags	• Recycling center
*Paint	• Donate • City hazardous waste collection
Paper, not mixed (white and colored, computer)	• Cut up and use for scrap paper, if possible • Recycling bin
Paper, mixed (metallic, carbon, and blueprints)	• Recycling center (check to see if they will accept before putting it in trash bin) • Trash bin
Paper bags	• Recycling bin
*Pesticides	• City hazardous waste collection
Phone books	• Recycling bin
Plastic bags (only clean plastic bags from shopping, newspaper coverings, bread bags, inside cereal boxes—you name it!)	• Either recycling bin (if allowed—often wrapped together in a tied-up plastic bag so that they won't fly loose), directly to the recycling center, or to a special recycling bin at your local grocery store—consult your local municipality or the administrator of the special recycling bin

Asterisked items are considered hazardous waste

(continued)

Type of Waste	Where to Dispose of It
Plastic bags *(continued)*	• It is important to send only clean plastic bags to recycling, because there is currently an issue with the nonrecyclability of soiled plastic bags, such as those with food particles adhering to them
Plastic containers (bottles, and food and beverage containers)	• Recycling bin (most municipalities will now take all plastics coded 1–7)
Plastic furniture	• Recycling center
Plastic shipping and packing material	• Recycling center (or a special recycling bin for plastic bags at your local grocery store—consult your local municipality)
*Pool chemicals	• City hazardous waste collection
Printer ink and toner cartridges	• Recycling center • Staples stores give store credit for bringing in used ink cartridges (www.staples.com)
Printers	• Recycling center
Remodeling waste (used kitchen countertops and cabinets)	• Donate, for example to an organization connected with the Reuse Development Corporation (www.redo.org) • Recycling center (if acceptable; if not, then the last resort is the trash bin)
*Shoe polish	• City hazardous waste collection
Shoes	• Recycling center • Donate
Styrofoam-like materials (packaging peanuts, cups, disposable dinnerware, and clamshell containers)	• Public drop-off collection site • Trash bin *Note: Few places recycle this poly-styrene (PS) product—best not to purchase it or frequent establishments that use it.*
Telephones	• Recycling center
*Thermometers that contain mercury	• City hazardous waste collection

Asterisked items are considered hazardous waste

Type of Waste	Where to Dispose of It
*Tires	• City hazardous waste collection
VHS tapes	• Recycling center

Asterisked items are considered hazardous waste

make recycling work

Here's what those recycling symbols mean:

  Universal recycling symbols indicate the product can be recycled.

 Universal recycling symbol encased within a dark circle means the product was *manufactured* with some already recycled materials.

 Universal recycling symbol encased within a dark circle *with a number* means the product was manufactured with a certain percentage of already recycled materials.

PETE

Plastic containers or bottles with the #1 code are the most widely used and recycled plastic and often have redemption value. PETE stands for polyethylene terephthalate. And the "phthalate" in terephthalate is different than the harmful phthalates found in other plastics and is not associated with phthalate leaching.

HDPE

Higher-density plastic containers or bottles that are recyclable and have the #2 code are often used for liquids like detergents or milk. HDPE means high-density polyethylene.

V

The label with the #3 code is for PVC plastic (thus the "V" under the number 3), which includes pipes, shrink wrap, plastic bags, bottles, and containers that are recyclable. PVC is dangerous to your health and the environment. PVC stands for polyvinyl chloride.

LDPE

The #4 code is for low-density plastic that can be recycled, including plastic bags, dry cleaning bags, trash can liners, and containers. Plastic bags can be dropped off at designated drop-off centers if your city recycling bin does not accept plastic bags. LDPE stands for low-density polyethylene.

PP

The #5 code is for a type of plastic that is often used for bottle caps, drinking straws, general food containers, and medicine containers. PP means polypropylene.

PS

The #6 code is for polystyrene (PS) plastic—most commonly referred to as Styrofoam. It is very costly and difficult to recycle.

OTHER

The #7 code is the category for any other type of plastic not covered by the previous six codes, including fiberglass, nylon, acrylic, and mixed plastics (such as products that have combined a plastic #1 and #4 into the same product). Additionally, polycarbonate is also a #7 plastic and should be avoided for any food use, as chemicals can leach from this type of polycarbonate plastic into a food or beverage.

styrofoam has got to go

Polystyrene plastic (PS), commonly referred to as Styrofoam, is a huge problem for our waste stream. Once manufactured, it is essentially nonbiodegradable. Styrofoam containers are usually used for food, and once the containers are contaminated, they cannot be recycled. As a result, it only takes a few minutes of use to create millions of years of nonbiodegradable debris. Additionally, PS is lightweight and often blows away during the trash collection process, ending up in the environment—on land or water—and harming animals.

On top of food use, PS is often found in packaging materials—such as for your newest electronic gadgets. Since there is virtually no recycling program out there for PS, you end up throwing all those little pieces into your regular trash bin. In the end, it is simply better not to purchase PS or anything that packages with PS. Sometimes this is difficult to know ahead of time, but if you have the opportunity, ask a business establishment how they will be packaging your purchase—food or otherwise—and if you have a greener option, take the greener path. Food establishments can use non-PS packaging or completely biodegradable packaging like corn-based plates and clamshells, and there are paper-based and other types of plastics that can safely package your purchases.

aluminum's silver lining

Aluminum is used in so many ways in your life. Of course, there's aluminum cans for your beverages and aluminum foil, but aluminum is also used to build automobiles, food containers, roofs, windows, aluminum siding, doors, and a home's structural framing—and these are just a few of its many uses.

Although original aluminum is mined and takes a lot of electricity to turn it into a usable metal, the good news is that aluminum is 100 percent recyclable. And it can be recycled an endless amount of times without compromising the integrity of the products in which it is used.

Additionally, when aluminum is recycled, it only uses 5 percent of the original energy used to make it from the mine. This means that aluminum is efficient and cost-effective to recycle, not to mention it is a durable metal. About 30 percent of the aluminum in the United States comes from recycled sources, so that means there's a lot of opportunity to improve. Take care to make sure that your aluminum can or any other product containing aluminum gets a chance to be recycled.

Look for Creative Ways to Reuse ☺ ✿

When you have children, nonhazardous household waste has many uses. Creative minds can turn trash into original crafts with a little glue, paint, markers, and crayons. You can also try these tips:

- Let your child play in any new big appliance or electronics box that comes into your home. It should get at least a couple weeks' worth of being a spaceship, before it goes into your recycling bin.
- Make gift tags by cutting up greeting cards and using a hole puncher and cotton string.
- Make homemade jigsaw puzzles by cutting up the fronts or backs of your cereal boxes.
- Make puppets out of old socks and fabric scraps (these scraps can come from old clothes).
- As long as there aren't any sharp edges, your child can build a playhouse for his toys out of used, cleaned food containers and boxes.

Consider a Compost ✚ ☺ $-$$

Of all the green ideas in this book, composting might very well be one of the hardest to get your family to buy into. Some people think it's gross or something Birkenstock-wearing hippies do, but composting is simply another way to recycle, and it's the way of the future. According to the EPA, 24 percent of America's solid waste comes from compostable yard trimmings and food waste.

At-home composting means recycling your food waste and some or all of your yard trimmings into something usable: a free nontoxic fertilizer, soil amendment, and mulch for your plants. Soil amendments and mulch help soil hold more water so that less irrigation is needed; keeps weeds down; controls erosion; and makes healthier plants and roots.

Additionally, composting is a more eco-friendly alternative to using a garbage disposal unit, which sends discarded food into the waste stream. And if you have a septic tank, a composting program can also decrease your tank's solids, reducing maintenance problems. If you live in an apartment, you can put composted material in patio plants, indoor potted plants, and in common green areas. For homes and condos with their own outdoor property, you have the option of sprinkling compost around your plants, trees, shrubs, and on your grass.

You can either compost using an outdoor composter or you can purchase an indoor kitchen composting device. Indoor composting devices will most likely not use bugs or worms, so you have the added advantage of being able to use the resulting compost in your indoor plants (bug free!) as well as outdoors. Some cities will even provide you with a free outdoor composter to encourage composting and to keep more waste out of the city's collection services. I'm fortunate that my city has one of the most progressive recycling centers in the nation and provides a free outdoor compost "machine" to residents, as well as composting information. In any case, you put your food waste (no bones, meats, or fats) into the compost instead of the trash bin and it breaks down, creating all-natural, nontoxic fertilizer and mulch. Surprisingly, it doesn't really take much time at all to compost once you set it up (and the initial setup only takes fifteen to thirty minutes of your time).

>> If you are composting, there should be very little going down your garbage disposal. This is better for improving your water supply since your municipal water treatment center has less dirty water to treat.

how to compost

Here's how to start an outdoor compost (and if you don't have an outdoor space, look into getting an indoor composter):

1. Contact your city's sanitation department to see if there is a composting program available. Be sure to inquire about educational workshops that might be offered, as well as whether

or not a free composter is given to residents. If your city doesn't offer free composters, check online or at your local garden center.

2. Put the composter in a place in your backyard, on soil (not concrete), that is, ideally, not too far from your kitchen. If you live in a warm climate, consider putting the composter near shade so the worms in the composter (they do the composting work) won't struggle with too much heat.

3. Fill up the composter with a *little* fresh dirt (half a shovel full) to start with and a few starter worms (only if you want, because worms will probably just come up from the soil under the compost anyway). After that, just start "cooking" your compost. The recipe is:

- *One part brown:* dried leaves, dried bread, coffee filters, paper napkins and towels, hair (from drains or your hairbrush), lint, small dried yard clippings, newspaper strips.
- *One part green:* food scraps from fruits, vegetables, eggshells, rice, and pasta; and green items like small just-cut plant trimmings, flowers, any vegetables or fruits that went bad on you and would otherwise be thrown away, and small amounts of grass.
- Add a little water, so that the compost is damp, but not soaked.
- Stir every week or two if you want it to cook faster (one to two months until done); do a little stirring if you want it to cook slower (three to six months until done). You can stir with a pitchfork, shovel, or any garden tool.
- If you adhere to this recipe, you can expect no offending smell.

4. You can collect food scraps in a closed pail under your kitchen sink. Or you can put a little bowl next to the side of the sink to collect items from each meal, and then when you clean up the kitchen just put those scraps in a newspaper-lined reusable container in the freezer (no rotting, no flies, no smell) or a plastic bag; when that freezer container is full, you dump it out in the composter (along with any newspaper liner) and some dried leaves. Easy.

5. Save dried leaves to cover up your green waste and to keep the flies away.

6. When the compost looks like black soil—some people call it "black gold"—shovel out the finished compost (sometimes from a door at the bottom, which is where the most finished compost will likely be) and sprinkle it on your lawn, around your shrubs and trees, and in your garden. It's free fertilizer, teeming with nutrients—and bugs and worms.

7. Don't be scared of the bugs and worms that will appear with any *outdoor* compost. This is how nature works. Worms and bugs in the compost are all part of the mini-ecosystem that made your black gold. They are excellent additions to your landscape—so don't pick them out!

BIO BAG >> (www.biobagusa.com) Sells a food collection system for composting.

EM AMERICA >> (www.emamerica.com) Has a product that can accelerate the composting process and help control odor in your outdoor composting area.

NATUREMILL >> (www.naturemill.com) Compact, in-the-kitchen composting machine that requires no worms or bugs to compost. This is a no-odor, heat-driven machine that gives you fresh compost for your houseplants, outdoor pots, or garden every two weeks, and because the composter works differently than an outdoor one, you can even compost dairy, meat, and fish.

THE EARTH MACHINE >> (www.earthmachine.com) Easy outdoor composter system—if you have a backyard—that is often provided to residents by local governments for free (contact your local sanitation department to see if this brand or other composter systems are available). The Earth Machine's Web site has lots of simple info on how to compost. You can also purchase this brand through online vendors such as www.composters.com.

Don't Pollute Your Household Water ✚

There are a number of things you should not put down your drain—neither the sink nor the toilet—to avoid contaminating the waste stream.

- Do not flush garbage down the toilet, as this causes added strain on your municipality's sewage system.
- Do not flush or pour hazardous waste down your toilet or drain. In general, this is anything labeled flammable, corrosive, an irritant, toxic, or poisonous. This includes paint, pesticides, herbicides, fertilizers, leftover cleaners, disinfectants, fuel, medications, nail polish remover or acetone, and pool chemicals. Unfortunately, many household cleaners—even toilet bowl cleaners—are really considered hazardous waste. So try to switch to nonhazardous cleaners.
- Avoid installing any kind of automatic water softening system. Some communities have completely banned traditional water softeners because of the way they pollute water. These systems use sodium chloride or potassium chloride to soften the water, and these compounds end up in the wastewater system and later in our rivers, crop fields, and oceans—harming agriculture, wildlife, and aquatic life. If your water is not too hard, then avoid a water softener altogether. Otherwise, look into a reverse osmosis system or a water softener system that does not discharge back into the sewer system and has, instead, a tank that a service periodically picks up and replaces. This is often called a portable exchange service where a softener's discharge is picked up and taken to an authorized receiver.

PURE-O-FLOW >> (www.pureoflow.com) This is a reverse osmosis system that purifies the water and removes hardness salts so that you get softer water without the chemicals.

LIFESTYLE ACTION

clean with care

what you need to know

The use of chemicals for cleaning has become commonplace in today's modern world, but many of them are toxic and are irritants, are not good for your health, and definitely strain your municipality's wastewater treatment system. In fact, the EPA has long had concerns about chemicals in cleaning products, as some cause reproductive disorders, organ damage, eye damage, headaches, dizziness, and fatigue. As a result, it is important to learn how to make less toxic cleaning decisions so that you clean in more earth-friendly and health-promoting ways.

Many greener cleaners can improve your indoor air quality and reduce potential health problems related to cleaning products, as well as be good for the environment—while still doing the cleaning jobs you need to have done. Unfortunately, there are a lot of unknowns with cleaning products, including the fact that manufacturers are not required to list all the ingredients, so you really have to educate yourself on how to read labels and know what you're looking for if you are going to make more environmentally sound and better-for-your-health purchasing and use decisions. In addition to household cleaners, many traditional cleaning practices also use a lot of energy and water that isn't always necessary.

benefits

By changing your cleaning products to nontoxic options and incorporating more energy- and water-efficient practices, you can improve the health of your family and the environment, as well as add money to your pocketbook.

how-to's

Do a Home Cleaning Supply Audit ✚

The first thing you can do to clean your home with care is to take inventory of your household cleaning products to determine what you have on hand and if any of the products are toxic. Many marketers are taking advantage of using keywords like "green" and "natural" on their products' labels, but you have to be a smarter consumer to really know if those words mean anything.

DO-IT-YOURSELF HOME CLEANING SUPPLY AUDIT	
Steps to Creating a Nontoxic Cleaning Product Supply	Completed
1. Gather up all home cleaning supplies.	
2. Review the product labels: • Take note of which products list all the ingredients (see page 97) and are detailed about what the product does, along with any claimed "eco" or "green" benefits. • You can further review product details by reading the product's Material Safety Data Sheet (MSDS) at the National Institutes of Health's online Household Products Database at http://householdproducts.nlm.nih.gov. The MSDS is your best source for understanding chemicals and what they mean for you and your family, especially since chemical listings can be so complex. • You can also go to any product's listed Web site to learn more about it, gain more ingredient details, and sometimes pull up an MSDS link if offered.	
3. Sort products into two piles: • Good—those that offer you full disclosure on ingredients. • Questionable—those that don't.	
4. Read the details of the products' labels—from the good pile see if there are any of these ingredients or keywords on the list; if yes, move to the questionable pile. • Any hazardous notes in the product's MSDS. • Products labeled with the words "corrosive," "toxic," "danger," or "caution." • Products with lye, hydrochloric acid, phosphoric acid, sulfuric acid, chlorine bleach, ammonia and ammonium compounds, phosphates, EDTA, petroleum, diethylene glycol, nonylphenol ethoxylate, butyl cellosolve, monoethanolamine (MEA), alkylphenol ethoxylates (APEs), paraffin, mineral oil, perchloroethylene, antibacterial agents like triclosan and benzalkonium chloride and phthalates.*	

*Not an all-inclusive list

Steps to Creating a Nontoxic Cleaning Product Supply	Completed
• Products with any indication of toxic VOCs. Usually the only indication you will have that there are VOCs in the product is that the product does not say "no VOC" or "low VOC." VOCs directly pollute your air (and form health hazards including carcinogenic hazards) or indirectly pollute your air by combining with ground-level ozone to form more hazardous air pollution. Ground-level ozone can be present indoors and outdoors. Examples of VOCs that directly pollute are alcohol, methanol, isopropanol, mineral spirits, glycol ethers, and formaldehyde. VOCs that indirectly pollute are primarily derived from strong plant oils and are called terpenes; these are mainly found in products that have citrus or pine ingredients as well as in air fresheners. • Any strong-smelling product. Strong smells may be an indication of having harmful VOCs or other hazardous and air-polluting elements. Sometimes companies will also use a strong-smelling fragrance to mask other odors from hazardous chemicals used in a cleaning product.	
5. Take note of the products that you have in the questionable pile: • Make a list of what you use them for. • Discard them according to the hazardous waste guidelines of your municipality. • Look for truly green alternatives to restock your cleaning supplies.	
6. Review your good pile: Look for additional labeling that gives you trust in the product—reviewing the company's Web site if necessary—otherwise discard and follow the steps in number 5. Green labeling to look for when keeping or purchasing cleaning products: • *Complete ingredient list.* Ideally this appears on the product's label. If not, you should be able to go online and get an MSDS to see everything about what is in the product. Many of the MSDS sheets will also list a score called HMIS Hazardous Material Information System, or HMIS. You want the score to be no higher than a 2. • *Third-party certification or label.* Examples include Green Seal, EcoLogo, or Design for the Environment (DfE). • *Sodium carbonate, sodium bicarbonate, sodium citrate, and sodium silicate.* According to the Union of Concerned Scientists, "these compounds work like phosphates and EDTA to soften water, but without the harmful impact." • *Nonchlorine bleach.* Without the hazard of chlorine, you can still whiten and brighten.	

(continued)

Steps to Creating a Nontoxic Cleaning Product Supply	Completed
• *Fragrance-free.* Many people are allergic to or irritated by fragrances, even if they are plant based. And when a product has no fragrance, the possibility of VOCs is reduced. • *No or low VOCs.* The label may state that there are no or low VOC emissions, including urea formaldehyde-free, CFC-free, HCFC-free, or halon-free.	

Avoid Harmful Chemicals ✚

In the Do-It-Yourself Home Cleaning Supply Audit I have listed a number of harmful chemicals to avoid. Here are some additional notes to be aware of:

• Avoid petroleum, which can come in the form of paraffin, mineral oil, diethylene glycol, perchloroethylene, butyl cellosolve, and nonylphenol ethoxylate. Petroleum is not only a nonrenewable resource but also its manufacturing pollutes your water and air.

• Avoid phosphates/EDTA, which are often found in dishwashing detergents, among other cleaning products. Choose the lowest phosphate level you can, because although phosphates (and their common alternative EDTA) soften water to make detergents work better, they aren't a good thing to have in your wastewater and there are healthier options. Once phosphates get in the wastewater they encourage algae growth, which can cut off oxygen for marine life. And EDTAs generally don't biodegrade, harming the skin and mucous membranes of marine life and later humans as it can reenter our water supply.

• Avoid phthalates, which are used in products that have scents so that the scents last longer. Phthalates are believed to cause cancer and reproductive diseases.

• Avoid antibacterial, found in lots of products out there. It is better to not choose antibacterial because of the potential danger of it causing antibiotic-resistant bacteria that could result in a superbug in humans that would be very difficult to treat.

- Avoid chlorine, which is often used for whitening and disinfecting. It is harmful to our water in large amounts, pollutes our air, and damages the earth's ozone layer.
- Avoid ammonia, which irritates your eyes and lungs. And if you have asthma or another lung malady, it can be a health risk.

>> Children inhale 50 percent more air per pound of body weight than adults, which makes them more sensitive to air quality problems, including chemicals from household cleaners that might be in the air. Additionally, babies and toddlers discover the world largely by touching and tasting—so they are more vulnerable to toxic residue from household cleaning.

it's in the small type

Some household cleaning products will give you a list of ingredients, but if you really look at the list, it's not a full disclosure about the actual ingredients. Complete disclosure can help you find harmful chemicals and lets you know which brands to trust for future shopping.

For example, let's take the All-Purpose "Green" Cleaner.

Ingredients on the Label
- Plant-derived surfactants (for soil removal)
- Natural alkalinity builder for enhanced performance (sodium citrate and sodium carbonate)
- Preservative (less than 0.05 precent)
- Water

Other Safety Features and Product Benefits on the Label
- Nontoxic
- Biodegradable
- No harsh chemicals
- No petroleum based solvents
- Multipurpose
- Heavy-duty
- No glycol ethers

- No phosphates
- No strong acids
- Not caustic
- No dyes
- No fragrances
- Not tested on animals

Label Analysis

- Unfortunately, there is only one actual ingredient listed—water
- By going to the company's Web site, however, the product's MSDS gives you a *complete* and *full* list of ingredients, although the complete list would have been better up-front on the package label.
- Additional important key words are on the label, like nontoxic and biodegradable.
- Although many green companies might claim a product is biodegradable, what is really important is how long it takes for the product to biodegrade *completely.* Three days? Or a hundred years? Better labeling will tell you up-front without having to ask.

terms to know: surfactants and solvents

A surfactant is basically a detergent that allows water to interact with oil and grease so they can be loosened, removed, and then pulled into the soapy or rinse water. Surfactants are foaming agents and can be made from petrochemicals or from plants or animals. All-purpose cleaners will contain some type of surfactant.

Solvents boost cleaning power so that you can be less abrasive and still get the job done. Solvents can be organic (like alcohol) or inorganic (like water) and they dissolve, extract, or suspend other materials from an object without changing or hurting the object or the solvent in the process—basically they clean with the intent of not leaving a residue. For example, when cleaning glass or removing fingerprints from walls, you want to clean the glass or walls but not leave cleaning marks behind.

Stock Up with Healthier Cleaning Products ✚ $–$$

Healthier cleaning products for you and your family are also better choices for the environment. The best cleaning product choices are:

- Made by yourself—that way you know what ingredients go into them.
- Purchased from companies who are dedicated to the development of truly eco-friendly cleaning products, who list their ingredients, whose MSDSs don't give you cause for concern, and who are actively seeking or who have obtained meaningful green seals of certification.

There are many cheap household ingredients that when combined make excellent, easy cleaners that do not harm your health nor the environment. These include: baking soda, distilled white vinegar, lemon juice, washing soda, and plain water. Also, in the past several years, a number of companies have sprung up that offer wide distribution of their eco-friendly cleaning products—Seventh Generation is one example.

mopping up excellence

Right now, there is not one seal of approval, like Energy Star or WaterSense, for household products, especially household cleaners. There is no U.S. law that requires manufacturers to list all ingredients, therefore it becomes more of a manufacturer's voluntary effort to list ingredients and seek certifications. There are also some useless "seals" of approval out there that are made by bogus nonprofit organizations; so make sure that any certification or label has numerous separate companies that it has certified products for before concluding the certification is real. And besides a label or seal of approval, be diligent about reading labels and making sure all the ingredients are listed—no seal can yet take the place of research on your part.

Currently there are three types of green certifications that include household cleaners, which can offer you some assistance in selecting green cleaning products. They are the Green Seal, the EcoLogo seal, and the Design for the Environment seal by the EPA.

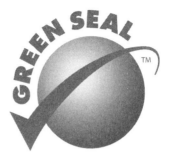

Green Seal (www.greenseal.org) is both the name of a nonprofit organization and its certifying label—the Green Seal. The seal means that a product is environmentally preferable over other products in its category.

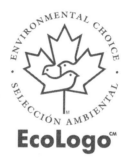

The EcoLogo (www.ecologo.org) certification is another green-type seal of approval that you can look for on products found in both the United States and Canada. The third-party program certifies products in more than 120 categories, including cleaning products.

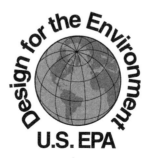

The Design for the Environment label (also called the DfE label) is an emerging certification and label promoted by the EPA (www.epa.gov/oppt/dfe). The label's purpose is to help consumers to quickly identify and choose products that can help protect the environment and are safer for families. In order to obtain the label, a manufacturer has to have all of the product's ingredients disclosed and evaluated.

ARM & HAMMER >> (www.armhammer.com) Baking soda and washing soda.

BIO BAG >> (www.biobagusa.com) Trash bags and shopping bags that are 100 percent biodegradable and 100 percent compostable.

BIOKLEEN >> (www.biokleenhome.com) Extensive line of biodegradable, concentrated, and nontoxic cleaning products, including eco-friendly carpet and rug shampoo and a fragrance-free line.

THE CLEANERSOLUTIONS DATABASE >> (www.cleaner solutions.org) A resource for you to determine the greenness and safety of cleaning products. You can sort the data by what you want to clean and by safety scores—the higher the safety score, the better. You can also search by company and product name.

DROPPS >> (www.dropps.com) Super-concentrated, eco-friendly laundry detergent that does not harm your clothes, your health, or the environment. Dropps also reduces waste by selling the product without a bottle or cap to recycle—the product comes in dissolvable packs that are equally as effective in cold water.

ECOVER >> (www.ecover.com) Full line of eco-friendly household cleaning products, which list ingredients.

GREEN WORKS >> (www.greenworkscleaners.com) Green cleaning products, including all-purpose cleaner, toilet bowl cleaner, and bathroom cleaner.

METHOD >> (www.methodhome.com) Green cleaning and household products, including a biodegradable and nontoxic daily shower spray that dissolves soap scum and mildew, several recognized by the Design for the Environment program.

PLANET >> (www.planetinc.com) Certified biodegradable cleaners and detergents.

SEVENTH GENERATION >> (www.seventhgeneration.com) Excellent line of green cleaning products, including dishwashing and laundry detergents, with full disclosure of ingredients, as well as eco-friendly paper and trash products like paper towels and recycled plastic trash bags.

SIMPLE GREEN >> (www.simplegreen.com) Many useful and widely available green-oriented cleaning products; on the company's Web site, a link to MSDSs for each product is available—excellent full disclosure.

STOUT >> (www.bettymills.com) Eco-friendly trash bag options.

Make Your Own Household Cleaning Products ✚ ☺ $

Although there's a little time and organization involved, you can make your own household cleaning products while saving yourself lots of money—and be greener and healthier in the process. Although the suggested mixtures have less hazardous ingredients than many commercial cleaners and pesticides, they should be used and stored with similar caution. Here's a list of some easy, do-it-yourself ways to clean green:

Household Cleaner Alternatives*

Drain cleaner: Use a plunger or plumber's snake. For sinks, undo the trap under the sink (the curved part of the pipe) to clean out a clog. You can also try a half cup of baking soda followed by one cup of distilled white vinegar, let bubble for fifteen minutes, then rinse with warm water. Some stubborn toilet clogs will need a plumber's attention.

Oven cleaner: Clean spills as soon as the oven cools using an all-purpose cream cleanser—even let cleanser soak in spills in the oven overnight; for tough stains, add salt (do not use this method in self-cleaning or continuous-cleaning ovens).

Glass cleaner: Mix one tablespoon of distilled white vinegar or lemon juice in one quart of water. Spray on glass and use newspaper to wipe dry.

All-purpose spray cleaner: One tablespoon washing soda with a squirt of liquid dishwashing soap and one quart of water.

All-purpose cream cleanser: Half cup baking soda and one tablespoon of liquid dishwashing soap (or until creamy).

Toilet bowl cleaner: Use a toilet brush and scrub with baking soda or distilled white vinegar. This will clean but not disinfect.

Furniture polish: Mix one teaspoon of lemon juice (or distilled white vinegar) in one tablespoon of vegetable oil (or olive oil), and wipe furniture. However, for general dusting, most furniture can just be wiped with a *damp* cloth—it's easier and fast.

Rug deodorizer: Deodorize dry carpets by sprinkling liberally with baking soda. Wait at least fifteen minutes and vacuum. Repeat if necessary.

---

*Compiled by author with information from the U.S. Environmental Protection Agency.

Silver polish: Boil two to three inches of water in a shallow pan with one teaspoon of salt, one teaspoon of baking soda, and a sheet of aluminum foil. Totally submerge silver and boil for two to three more minutes. Wipe away tarnish. Repeat if necessary. (Do not use this method on antique silver knives as the blade can separate from the handle.) Another alternative is to use nonabrasive toothpaste.

Plant cleaner: Wipe leaves with mild soap and water; rinse.

Mothballs: Use cedar chips, lavender flowers, rosemary, mint, or white peppercorns.

Flea and tick products: Put brewer's yeast or garlic in your pet's food; sprinkle fennel, rue, rosemary, or eucalyptus seeds or leaves around animal sleeping areas.

Air freshener: Open your window and let in fresh air; place baking soda in an open container to absorb odors; put a scented soy candle in a glass jar on a mug warmer (avoids having a burning flame); or add plants or fresh flowers, which help absorb chemicals and give off fresh, natural scents.

Laundry stain remover: One-fourth cup of baking soda and one-half cup of warm water to pretreat stains—check that the item is colorfast because baking soda can have a whitening effect.

Warning!
- DO NOT mix any of these ingredients with a commercial cleaning agent.
- Store all household cleaners away from children—even these homemade ones.
- If you store a homemade mixture, make sure it is *properly labeled* and do not store it in a container that could be mistaken for food or beverage.

- When preparing alternatives, mix only what is needed for the job at hand and mix them in clean, reusable containers. This avoids waste and the need to store any cleaning mixture.
- Washing soda is stronger than baking soda and can irritate your skin, so wear gloves.
- Purchase eco-friendly liquid dishwashing soap instead of the traditional type.

> **WOMEN'S VOICES FOR THE EARTH >>** (www.womenandenvironment.org) This women's environmental organization has a Host a Green Cleaning Party program where you and your friends get together to make your own nontoxic cleaning products.

clean your i.q.

We live with microscopic organisms, including germs, every day. According to the latest research, this isn't such a bad thing, since it helps to build up our immunity against disease. Unless you are in a hospital or have home health care for an immune-suppressed family member, you can stop worrying and just do average, smart cleaning to keep your family healthy. Here are some recommended guidelines:

Back off from antibacterial. There has been some controversy over whether or not antibacterial household cleaning and hygiene products might create antimicrobial drug resistance. While the U.S. Centers for Disease Control and Prevention (CDC) says this fear is currently inconclusive and requires more study, they also say there is no advantage found in using antibacterial products when compared to plain soap. I recommend you avoid the potential risks and extra expense and steer clear of all antibacterial products.

Wash your hands often. This is the number one way, according to the CDC, that you can prevent the spread of disease. Wash your hands with soap in hot running water for at least fifteen seconds before eating, after touching public spaces (handrails, shopping carts), after using the bathroom, after petting animals, after shaking people's hands, or after sneezing or coughing. Wait to touch your face until washing your hands after shaking hands or touching public spaces.

Use steam. You can get away with using no chemicals for your deeper cleaning with steam cleaner machines, which use just water vapor. They are extremely effective at disinfecting without any harmful chemicals.

Use your dishwasher. Your dishwasher is a safe alternative to disinfecting your dishes and cutting boards, and you can still choose an environmentally friendly dishwasher detergent without sacrificing the disinfecting, because it is largely the heat that disinfects.

Look for new green disinfectant products. Most green-labeled cleaning products will not claim to disinfect by themselves. However, there are essential or botanical oils—lavender oil being one of them—that have long traditions of being antibacterial, antifungal, and are biodegradable and ecologically safe.

As a last resort, use a conventional disinfectant cleaner. Although all the previous tips here should take care of most of your disinfecting needs, there are times when you might have special concerns about disinfecting for serious health reasons. In those cases, as an added health protection, you can use Clorox or Lysol brand disinfectants. They have been found to be the most effective against the most threatening of bacteria.

BISSELL >> (www.bissell.com) Has a steam mop that is easy to use. Read more about their green initiatives and eco-friendly products at www.getalittlegreen.com.

WHITEWING STEAMER >> (www.allergybuyersclubshopping .com) A steamer for cleaning that has a mop and other attachments to clean nearly all surfaces in your home.

white glove advice

Seventh Generation has been a leader in green cleaning since 1988. Martin Wolf, the company's director of product and environmental technology, says that washing thoroughly with a soap or detergent and water is usually sufficient to minimize the risk of infection from most household surfaces.

He says, "The Food and Drug Administration recently proposed banning antimicrobial hand soaps because there is no evidence that using these products is any more effective than using plain soap and water, and antimicrobial products carry a higher human health and environmental risk. Disinfectants, including antimicrobial or antibacterial hand soaps and products, often contain nondegradable chemicals called quaternary ammonium chlorides and chlorinated phenol compounds. Chlorinated phenol compounds are now known to be extremely toxic and persistent in the environment. Thus using an antimicrobial agent poses more risk than benefit."

If you want to disinfect for a particular reason, such as cleaning cutting boards or countertops after working with raw meat, or because of the recent illness of a family member, Wolf recommends that you go the all-natural route. Use gloves and protect your eyes. Spray the surface to be disinfected with vinegar; allow the surface to dry, or wipe with a clean sponge or towel after five minutes. This is an effective way to disinfect without some of the hazards associated with conventional antimicrobial/ antibacterial products or household chlorine bleach.

Clean with Reusable Supplies ☺ ✿

Whenever possible, look for ways to clean using reusable materials. This can save you money and conserve our planet's resources. For example, dry with a dish towel or air dry instead of using a paper towel. Or, clean with a rag or towel that can be washed. Shake out the dust or particles from your reusable towel into the garbage before washing. If you use paper towels, look for ones made from recycled content.

>> Fabric softener sheets are more eco-friendly. Reuse them after the dryer to dust your furniture.

>> When taking your car to be washed, look for commercial car washers that reuse (recycle) their water instead of using new water for every car.

Vacuum Using a HEPA Vacuum Cleaner ✚ $$

When you want to vacuum your floors for everyday cleanliness, look into getting a vacuum cleaner with a HEPA (High Efficiency Particle Arrestor) filter, which will filter out both large and microscopic particles like dust, pet dander (pet skin flakes), mold, smoke, pollen, and bacteria which can make you sick or trigger allergies. Read the HEPA filter's label before buying to make sure it is a quality filter—the label should state that the filter's test results show that it traps particles as small as .3 microns and will trap 99.97 percent or above in particles. A serial number will be listed on the package or the filter itself.

ARM & HAMMER >> (www.armhammervac.com) Has line of HEPA vacuum filters.

BISSELL >> (www.bissell.com) Sells several different types of HEPA-filtered vacuums.

DIRT DEVIL >> (www.dirtdevil.com) Sells HEPA vacuums, and many of their HEPA filters can be partially recycled.

ELECTROLUX >> (www.electrolux.com) HEPA vacuums with the added ability to trap particles in a sealed compartment.

HOOVER >> (www.hoover.com) Has HEPA vacuum cleaners.

Wash in Cold Water Whenever Possible ☺

Although you may have grown up thinking that all whites are washed with hot water and colors with cold, these notions are largely a by-product of appliance and detergent marketers who looked for ways to identify features and educate the public on ways to launder. Most of the time you only need to wash your clothes in cold water unless they are quite dirty or need sanitizing. I almost always wash in cold water because our clothes are not really that soiled. The hotter the water, the more cleaning action it can give—removing germs and heavy dirt.

Even warm water can take more of a toll on your clothes than cold water—causing them to possibly shrink, wrinkle, and fade. This is why delicate items need cold water, not hot. Cold water also saves you from paying to heat up your water, plus it makes your clothes last and look better longer. Use cold water to pretreat or soak stained items. If your current detergent isn't properly dissolving or cleaning well in the cold water, look for another eco-friendly option that is specifically formulated for cold water.

Cut Down on Power Drying ☺ ✿ $-$$$

Traditional dryers not only use lots of electricity but also cause wear and tear on your clothes. Fortunately, there are now new-generation Energy Star-rated dryers with moisture sensors and other technologies that dry clothes using less energy. A moisture sensor detects when your clothes are dry and then automatically powers down the drying cycle and turns off the machine. If you live in a fairly dust-free climate, consider the option of drying clothes outdoors and on drying racks.

Don't forget to clean out the lint catcher in the dryer each time you dry your clothes. This will help to boost your dryer's energy efficiency. Once or twice a year clean out the vent that goes from your dryer to the outside—this will keep your drying safe by preventing a potential fire and the dryer running at peak efficiency.

Look into Eco-Friendly Dry Cleaning ✚

We all want our clothes to look great, but traditional dry cleaning methods use a dry cleaning solvent called perchloroethylene (PERC or PCE), also called tetrachloroethylene or tetrachlorethylene. This chemical can cause serious health problems with long-term exposure, including neurological, liver, kidney, and reproductive damage; along with a potential higher risk for cancer. It also is a hazardous substance to dispose of, which is not eco-friendly to us or to the earth.

According to the National Institutes of Health, you can be exposed to this chemical if you dry clean your clothes. After your clothes are cleaned, they can release small amounts of perchloroethylene into the air. You can also be exposed if you use a Laundromat that contains dry cleaning machines. Perchloroethylene is also in products such as fabric finishers, adhesives, spot removers, typewriter correction fluid, shoe polish, and wood cleaners.

Short-term exposure to low levels of perchloroethylene can cause dizziness, inebriation, and sleepiness; and can irritate eyes, nose, mouth, throat, and the respiratory tract. Direct contact with perchloroethylene liquid or vapor can irritate and burn the skin, eyes, mouth, and throat. Some dry cleaners have started using silicon as a dry cleaning solvent and calling it "green" dry cleaning, but there is some question as to whether that method is actually environmentally friendly.

Instead of dry cleaning, see if it is possible to hand wash the clothes that you would normally take to the cleaners. Otherwise, seek out a more eco-friendly dry cleaning service that does not use PERC or silicone. Most will actively promote their greenness—and will probably be using carbon dioxide or wet cleaning. If you do not have an eco-friendly dry cleaner nearby or if they're cost-prohibitive, then be sure to air out your clothes after you bring them back from a traditional dry cleaner, preferably in a place where you won't be breathing in any release of fumes left over from the cleaning process.

> >> Since many dry cleaning supplies such as garment covers, garment bags, hangers, and pins are often not accepted in your municipality's recycling bin, ask your dry cleaner if they will take them back for recycling.

dry cleaning revealed

The Pollution Prevention Center at the Urban and Environmental Policy Institute of Occidental College in Los Angeles is actively promoting public awareness of better choices when it comes to your dry cleaning.

Peter Sinsheimer, the center's director, says, "Most dry cleaners worldwide use the toxic chemical perchloroethylene (PCE) as the cleaning solvent. PCE is a probable human carcinogen, a neurotoxin, and a hazardous air pollutant."

However, there are now two viable environmentally friendly alternatives that some cleaners are using—water-based professional wet cleaning and CO_2 dry cleaning (which uses recycled carbon dioxide). Professional wet cleaning is extremely energy efficient and saves water as well. Through California laws, PCE is being phased out and the state encourages dry cleaners to switch to wet cleaning and CO_2.

"If people don't have a CO_2 or wet cleaning near them they should ask their cleaner about at least adding wet cleaning. Our studies show that for cleaners who need to replace their dry cleaning machine, the operating cost in wet cleaning is actually lower than for dry cleaning," says Sinsheimer.

Alternatives to traditional dry cleaning:

 • Wet cleaning is nontoxic, energy efficient, and environmentally friendly. Most garments labeled "dry clean only" can be professionally wet cleaned. Recent studies on this technology show that wet cleaning is comparable to dry cleaning in quality, price, and turnaround time.

• CO_2 cleaning uses an industrial by-product from existing operations. Since it does not produce any new CO_2, it does not contribute to global warming.

FINDCO2.COM >> (www.findco2.com) This Web site helps you find a CO_2 dry cleaner near you.

your green garden: add to the health and safety of your outdoors

Your garden—whether a simple houseplant, some herbs on your windowsill, fruits and vegetables in the backyard, or a verdant field blooming with life in all seasons—no doubt brings you joy and beauty. Return the favor by using a truly *green* thumb when caring for it.

LIFESTYLE ACTION

create an eco-friendly garden

what you need to know

About 83 percent of American households do some type of lawn or garden project every year. This is good news, as it means we're not always in our car or inside watching TV. Gardening is not only a popular pastime but also a property necessity. Plants add beauty to your environment; give you sensory pleasure with their beauty, colors, and scents; and play an important role in providing you with clean air and the needed nutrition you get from the food you eat.

Additionally, how you take care of your lawn, garden, and plants affects the air around your home and in your community, adds or detracts from your natural and local wildlife and ecosystems, affects your local and regional water supply, and influences your mental health.

Unfortunately, many of us have not taken care of our lawns and gardens in an eco-friendly way. This has resulted in large amounts of pesticides, herbicides, and fertilizers in our waterways, which flow to and pollute our oceans. The Ocean Project (www.theoceanproject .org), an ocean conservation group, says that more than 70 million pounds of toxic lawn pesticides are applied annually in the United States alone—much of it flowing off the land via rain and irrigation and later ending up in rivers and oceans, harming aquatic and ocean life. Because of this toxic runoff (also caused by industrial and agricultural waste) there are now coastal dead zones where no animals can survive. Additionally, land-based wildlife and insects, not to mention humans, come in contact with toxic pesticides on plants and in the soil and streams. In fact, according to the American Bird Conservancy, 67 million birds die every year because of the toxic effects of pesticides.

Every household must contribute to the health of our ecosystems, because eventually unhealthy ecosystems and their polluted habitats will affect us by either making us sick or by not providing us with much needed food and nutrients. This will become a frightening reality unless everyone—consumers and businesses worldwide—behaves more responsibly towards our earth.

benefits

Healthy garden practices have many immediate and long-term benefits, including improving your air (indoor and out), boosting your mood, increasing your property value, providing you with nutritious and organic food, and helping the surrounding and regional ecosystem's health and sustainability.

how-to's

Plant Trees ☺ ✚ $-$$$$

As I mentioned in chapter 1, there are a multitude of economic and habitat-preservation reasons for planting trees, but there are also mental health benefits. Trees, and other greenscape, help to boost your brain power and reduce your stress.

>> Cornell University has done research on the effect of plants, trees, green lawns, and other greenscape and how it affects your mental health, and the conclusions are significant. Researchers found that when a child's home was surrounded by nature, it helped to boost attention span and brain function, lower stress levels, and improve psychological well-being.

Try a Container Garden ☺ ✚ ✿ $–$$

Whether you have a backyard, patio, or just a windowsill, you can still have a garden. Just think small! No matter how limited your time or small your budget, you can dig your hands into the dirt with a container garden. Container gardening is simply that—planting a little garden (or just one plant!) inside some type of container. Here are some items conducive to container gardening:

- Flowers
- Herbs
- Vegetables
- Houseplants
- Succulents
- Trees

how to choose container trees

You have to do your research when considering a container tree, since not all trees are suited to growing in such a small space. Ask your local nursery for suggestions. Here are some tips:

- For outdoor containers, look for native tree varieties that will benefit local pollinators and wildlife.
- Choose a tree based on how much sunshine and heat it will receive.
- Purchase or make a container—most need to be at least two feet in diameter—that has drainage so that the roots will not be sitting in undrained water.
- Many dwarf varieties are excellent for containers.

- Ask your nursery if the tree's root system will allow for growth in a constricted space.
- Learn how to trim and prune the tree—including any root pruning—to control its size and promote its good health.

Create a Pollinator Garden ✚ $–$$

According to the National Gardening Association, one out of every three bites of food that we eat comes from a plant that was pollinated—usually either by bees, bats, wasps, butterflies, beetles, birds, moths, lizards, or flies. In fact, 80 percent of all plants that flower—including many flowering trees that produce nuts and fruits and flowering vegetables—require pollination in order to successfully survive.

Unfortunately the overuse of pesticides, as well as other factors, has weakened pollinating species so that they have a harder time doing their job. In some cases, whole colonies of species have mysteriously collapsed. As a result, if pollinators—bees in particular—are not taken care of in a more eco-friendly way, our food supply could be in serious danger. You can do your part by creating a garden that can keep these pollinators happy and healthy throughout the various seasons.

Pollinator Garden How-To's

1. Reduce or eliminate pesticides and herbicides and look for alternatives.

2. Add flowers and flowering trees to your property's landscape—make sure you install a variety of species so that you have blooms at different times during the year to feed your pollinators.

- Use as many native varieties as possible, as these will be easier for the pollinators to adapt to.
- Hybrid or imported flowers or flowering plants are not always accepted by local pollinators.
- If there are night-blooming plants or trees in your garden, this can offer another option for nocturnal pollinators like bats, moths, or beetles.
- Vary colors, because some pollinators like yellow more than red,

or blue and purple more than orange and pink.

- Consider turning some of your property into a wildflower garden.
- Grow flowers in containers—offer a variety of herbs, annuals, and perennials.

3. Provide a water source. Although you don't want to breed mosquitoes, consider how much water is available near your property.

- Butterflies need water and bees and wasps need mud puddles for gathering building materials.
- If there is not much water nearby, add a birdbath.
- Allow some irrigated dirt to be exposed here and there to form mud puddles in the morning hours from your morning watering.
- Add larger rocks with shallow depressions, which will fill up in the morning with the water from your sprinkler system but burn off by evening so that mosquitoes cannot breed in them.
- The Humane Society of the United States (www.hsus.org) recommends "a dish of wet sand or small inground sandy area" in a garden to encourage "puddling"—this is for butterflies so that they can gather to siphon up water and minerals.

"bee" right!

If you see a bee colony on your property or even in your home, don't have it destroyed! Natural and native pollinator colonies are very important to our food supply and the surrounding ecosystem. Instead, request that the colony be relocated by a bee specialist. Bee professionals will carefully remove the honeycomb (the bees' home) and relocate it to another area, such as a local farm that supports and embraces bee colonies.

Regrettably, too many pest exterminator companies will use hazardous pesticides to kill off a bee colony. This is not only inhumane but also harmful to the environment and to you and your family, who can come in contact with the pesticides. Plus, a pesticide kill off can result in a maggot infestation. The smell of dead, rotting bees and fermenting honey can be unbearable. Also, moths can feed off of the honeycomb and breed into a new problem.

Grow Healthy Produce ☺ ✚ $–$$

One way to insure the safety and health of your food is to grow it your-self. Unlike most of the foods in our stores, there won't be a question as to whether or not your produce was treated with pesticides, herbicides, or harmful fertilizers; plus you'll be able to pick it when it's ripe, allowing for the most amount of nutrients.

Let's be real, though—most of us do not have the land or the time to spend gardening all our meals. How much produce gardening you desire to do or can do is a matter of time and priorities. One easy way is through trees that produce fruit and nuts—especially ones that can wait on the tree for a time before you are ready to pick or use them, such as citrus varieties. Container gardening of herbs and vegetables is another option when space and time are issues.

One of the most important things when gardening for home produce is to know what seasons you should grow various items in for your par-ticular climate. Get free educational help from your local government. Experts at the Cooperative Extension System Office (www.csrees.usda .gov/Extension), which is run by the U.S. Department of Agriculture, can help teach you how to garden and what to garden in your area and cli-mate during the various seasons; there are local extension offices not far from most communities across the United States.

> >> When you start seedlings indoors, choose peat pots instead of plastic pots. A peat pot is biodegradable and gets planted with the seedling when it's ready to go outdoors.

kids have green thumbs, too

When it comes to being a green mom, gardening is one of the best ways to teach your children to love and protect the earth. Start gardening when they're young so you teach them to love nature from the get-go. Here are some ideas on how to involve your family in gardening:

Plant a seed in a cup, in a small container, or out in your garden—water it, give it sunlight, and watch it grow.

Trim and weed together: It gets the job done faster, plus everyone has an appreciation for the work done and beauty created.

Let your child create his or her own little garden and don't put too many limitations on the seeds sowed.

Purchase a package of ladybugs and have your children let them out into your garden.

Hang up a hummingbird or bird feeder near a window where your family can watch birds come and go.

Plant flower bulbs together, then watch them come up in their season.

Dig up a garden together that needs to start anew—kids love digging.

Let your child water the plants with a watering can on a hot day.

BALL FOOD STORAGE >> (www.freshpreserving.com) An informative Web site on how you can preserve your home produce.

Enrich Your Local Wildlife's Habitat ✚ $–$$

When you invest in the health and eco-friendliness of your landscape's habitat, you and your family will be able to not only enjoy the beauty it provides you, but also the opportunity to interact and sustain your local wildlife. Unfortunately, according to the Humane Society "wildlife habitat continues to be fragmented or eliminated at an alarming rate, leaving wild animals vulnerable to many dangers in our cities and towns—though we cannot undo our urban or suburban landscapes, we can find ways to make our shared spaces more hospitable to those wild creatures who have survived our changes to the landscape."

There are many things you can do to enrich your property for local wildlife. The National Wildlife Federation (www.nwf.org) recommends:

Provide food sources for wildlife: Install native plants that will supply seeds, fruits, nuts, berries, and nectar.

Provide water sources for wildlife: Add a birdbath, pond, and water garden; create or restore a stream.

Provide places for wildlife cover: Plant a thicket (dense growth of shrubs or underbrush), create a rock pile, or install a birdhouse.

Provide places for wildlife to raise its young: Set up dense shrubs, vegetation, a nesting box, or a pond.

Garden sustainably: Add mulch, compost, or use chemical-free fertilizer.

feed 'em the good stuff

Here are some tips for what to feed your wild birds, adapted from the Humane Society of the United States Web site:

Sunflower seeds: Usually attracts the greatest variety of birds, especially those that frequent trees and who prefer to perch while feeding. While hulled sunflower seeds are more expensive, they help reduce the mess when birds feed.

White proso millet seed: Popular for ground-feeding birds like doves and sparrows. The feeder should be mounted on a post one to two feet above the ground.

Do not overfill: Feeders should be filled with only enough seed to be consumed by the local birds in one to two days, otherwise the feeder could be contaminated by bird feces or could spread disease.

Avoid bargain-type bird seeds: Especially avoid mixed seeds. Most birds will just pick through until they reach the sunflower or millet seeds, leaving the others tossed on the ground to decompose.

Include a birdbath: Place it in your backyard or on the porch— birds will use it for drinking water and bathing year-round. Place the birdbath away from bird feeders so that bird droppings and seeds do not contaminate the water. The birdbath should be rinsed daily and kept at a shallow height of one to two inches.

no-bake suet cake

A fun fall or wintertime activity to do with kids is to make a suet cake for wild birds. It is a combination of fat (suet) and seeds or fruit that gives birds food and energy in the colder months. One simple way to make suet cake is to get a pinecone and put a mixture of one part peanut butter and five parts cornmeal into the cone's crevices and hang with a string from a tree branch. Your local bird club may also have other suet recipes for the birds in your area. (Don't put out a suet cake if the outside temperature is over eighty degrees because the fat may turn rancid.)

six steps to going wild

The National Wildlife Federation (www.nwf.org) has a fun family program called the Certified Wildlife Habitat program. It's a six-step process of making simple changes in your garden to help sustain local wildlife, and includes providing food, water, cover, and places to raise young. The program can help you attract interesting wildlife to view up close or from your window, such as songbirds, butterflies, and frogs. The beauty of your property is also increased by adding native wildflowers, trees, and shrubs. And you are also helping the overall environment in a fun way that kids love.

Eliminate Harmful Lawn Pesticides and Herbicides ☺ ✚ $

You might have a dream home with an enviable lawn and garden, but what lurks beneath it might another story—one of a toxic mess in the form of pesticides and herbicides.

Although we grew up using these products for our lawn and garden, the ugly truth is they not only harm the local ecosystem but also ecosystems miles away, pollute our waterways and oceans, kill wildlife and bees, and put our health and the health of our environment in peril. When you overuse a hose or sprinkler on your property, or whenever it rains, any runoff water goes down the drain into the storm water system. Everyone else's lawn is also draining off, including your local parks' and business' landscapes. All that runoff—along with motor oil and pet waste—combines to make a toxic soup that goes straight into your area's waterways or the ocean—untreated. Storm water in many areas is not treated because of the sheer volume of it. As a result, your gardening directly affects the health of your land and water and all the animals above and below ground as well as aquatic life.

The best thing you can do when it comes to pesticides and herbicides is reduce or eliminate their use. This reduction or elimination of pesticides and a focus on prevention is called integrated pest management, or IPM. Here are alternatives:

Learn to love some bugs: Many bugs are good for your lawn and garden, including earthworms, butterflies, moths, lacewings, bees, wasps, flies, ladybugs, centipedes, praying mantises, and many types of beetles.

Add ladybugs: Ladybugs (also called lady beetles) are such good little insects. They efficiently eat aphids and other plant-eating pests—one ladybug can eat up to 5,000 aphids in its lifetime. Your local garden center will likely sell live ladybugs.

Get rid of bad bugs the better way: Many people see a plant's partially eaten leaf and pull out the pesticide bottle. But plants are food to lots of critters and insects—it's natural. If you can see little bugs on the plants, try some water spraying. A few days of blasting the leaves with a hose should get rid of things like aphids and other small insect pests. You can also rid your garden of slugs with beer. Put a plate of beer on the ground and watch the slugs come in droves! They will drown in the liquid.

natural pest control

If you've tried ladybugs and hosing with water to no avail, then try this homemade nontoxic bug spray mix. (Protect your eyes!)

Mix in a spray bottle:

- ¼ cup eco-friendly liquid soap
- 2 tablespoons hot pepper sauce (the hottest you can find)
- 3 diced garlic cloves
- 1 cup water

You can spot spray as needed—but just as with any commercial pesticide, naturally made pesticides can also harm beneficial insects if you don't use restraint.

Other ideas:

Add strong-scented flowers, herbs, and plants: Lavender, marigold, rosemary, sweet basil, garlic, and onions are just a few examples of some of the excellent options you have when it comes to natural pest control. The strong scents from these plants confuse pests and drive them away.

Prevent weeds: Mulch stops a lot of unwanted weed growth. Set aside time to periodically weed—it's old-fashioned, but it works. Pull weeds out from the root. Mow higher, as this discourages weeds. For pesky lawn weeds that are just too difficult to get rid of by pulling, you can spot spray them with vinegar. But don't overdo it! A lot of vinegar in your soil isn't good. Another natural lawn approach is corn gluten meal as a weed suppressant. It is useful as a preemergent, not after the weeds have established. There is also a benefit to using this approach: It adds natural nitrogen as plant food for what you want to keep—your lawn.

ST. GABRIEL LABORATORIES >> (www.milkyspore.com) Offers a natural weed control (Premerge) made from corn gluten meal, and other eco-friendly lawn and garden products.

Go native: Native plants often need little pesticide usage since they resist most types of local disease, pests, and weather conditions without any human help. Plant them in an area that receives proper sunlight and provide some supplemental irrigation.

Avoid Diazinon: If you have any pesticide product in your home or garage that has the ingredient diazinon in it, you need to stop using it and take it to your city's hazardous waste collection drop-off. Diazinon has harmful effects on humans and birds.

Look for eco-friendly products: If you need to take more pest or weed action than the above, look for eco-friendly pest and weed control products which make an effort to list *all* the ingredients and provide you with access (usually online) to the MSDS to check out any hazards. Look for any third-party certifications on the label.

BEYOND PESTICIDES >> (www.beyondpesticides.org) Helpful nonprofit organization that provides useful information on pesticides and alternatives to their use.

GREEN SHIELD CERTIFIED >> (www.greenshieldcertified.org)
An independent, nonprofit certification program that has a directory of effective, prevention-based pest control providers who also
minimize the use of pesticides.

THE IPM INSTITUTE OF NORTH AMERICA >> (www.ipm
institute.org) This nonprofit organization is a great resource for
learning how to reduce pesticide use.

get rid of mosquitoes the smart way

If you have a mosquito problem, you should try to get rid of them and protect yourself with alternative measures other than insecticides or pesticides. One way to stop mosquitoes from breeding without using pesticides
is by preventing any standing water on your property. Check for trapped
water in old tires, buckets, and plant pots. Empty out your birdbath every
day so that mosquito eggs cannot take hold. And then if you need added
protection so you don't get bit, look for alternatives to DEET, which is a
chemical commonly found in conventional insect repellants but has been
found to cause skin, eye, and neurological problems. Ideas for alternatives:

Cover more of your skin: Try long pants and long shirts.

Spend more time behind screens: Such as a screened porch or
screened window.

Use yellow bug lights: Replace your outdoor porch lights with
antibug lights, which have a special yellow coating that don't
attract bugs; Feit Electric (www.feitelectric.com) has a yellow
antibug compact fluorescent light.

Use herbal insect repellants: For DEET-free options, try Bite
Blocker (www.biteblocker.com) which is made with soybean and

coconut oils, or Burt's Bees' (www.burtsbees.com) Herbal Insect Repellent.

Fertilize with Care ☺ ✚ $

Fertilizing is another area where the results might look great but the means to the end could be unhealthy for your soil, walkways, and surrounding wildlife. Here are some guidelines:

Water longer but less often: It is better to water for a longer period of time and less frequently to encourage stronger roots and plants.

Fertilize your lawn the least amount of times to get the green results you desire.

Look into time-release fertilizers or microdose fertilizing through your irrigation: Time-release options include slow-release granules and slow-release sticks that you push into the soil—a time-release approach allows the plants to absorb the nutrients over time and decreases the chance of fertilizers running off into the storm water or polluting ground water supplies. Another option is the release of microdoses of fertilizer through your irrigation system each time you water, which nearly eliminates fertilizer runoff (as long as your irrigation is set up properly) and which also ends up reducing water usage because of a healthier plant root system.

Use material from a compost to fertilize and amend your soil: This will make your soil retain moisture more easily, return needed nutrients to the soil, and strengthen plants without any toxicity.

Use clippings to fertilize: Lawn clippings, especially those that come from a mower that mulches, are free slow-releasing fertilizer for your lawn. Use some extra lawn clippings as fertilizer around other plants, too.

Look for organic fertilizers: If you buy fertilizers, seek out those made from organic matter instead of chemical ones—some examples are manure, compost, and agricultural by-products. However, organic fertilizers do not give you the license to fertilize more or irresponsibly—use sparingly.

>> Here's a nontoxic, organic, and inexpensive way to give your outdoor rose bushes some much-needed potassium nutrients—bury up to three banana peels per week in the soil around the bushes, and the decomposing peel will leach out potassium.

Apply at or after sundown: If you have a garden problem that must be addressed with a more hazardous pesticide or herbicide, apply at or after sundown when a good portion of the beneficial pollinators and bugs have completed their work for the day.

DR. BENSON'S NATURAL MIX >> (www.drbensonsmix.com) Natural fertilizer with no salts. Also safe for your organic produce garden.

EZ-FLO >> (www.ezfloinjection.com) Microdose fertilizer system done through your irrigation or sprinklers that results in much less fertilizer and water used and healthy plants.

NATURALAWN >> (www.nl-amer.com) Organic-based lawn care service with franchises throughout the United States.

Reduce Gardening Emissions ✚ $$–$$$

Mowers, blowers, and hedge trimmers—basically anything that runs on gas—have harmful emissions. So use a broom and a rake instead of a blower whenever possible. Consider switching to electric or lower-emission options for your other gardening machines.

STIHL >> (www.stihlusa.com) Sells backpack and electric blowers, trimmers, and chainsaws that have lower emissions engines, as well as nonpetroleum-based oils and lubricants that biodegrade in twenty-one days.

check out the greenscapes program

The EPA has formed a new certification program called GreenScapes (www.epa.gov/greenscapes). Through GreenScapes, you can learn more about maintaining an eco-friendly garden and lawn, as well as how to save money on water. The program also has useful resources on lawn and garden services and products that adhere to the GreenScape principles.

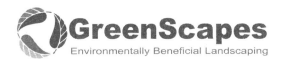

LIFESTYLE ACTION

make outdoor water count

what you need to know

There are few things more pleasant to look at and relax in than a lush, green landscape with flowers and trees. But for many areas a lush, green landscape isn't native—take Phoenix, Arizona, for example. I lived there for many years, and water conservation was on our family's minds and reflected in our landscape. We took advantage of native trees and plants and were able to create our own desert lushness—but this lushness included many cactus varieties.

Water-efficient native-plant gardens and landscapes pay homage to the environment in which they are grown. Furthermore, depending on where you live, water conservation for outdoor watering can be a big issue. In many areas of the western United States, where there isn't a lot of rain, more than half of the water bill might be for landscape needs. You need to be aware that the amount of water you use will have a major impact on the health of your plants, the availability of water in general, and your budget.

Additionally, urban water runoff can be a problem in many areas. This is when excess water from a storm or from irrigation runs off your property and into storm drains, and this water carries with it all the chemicals you have been using on your lawn and landscape into the local creeks, reservoirs, and ocean. This affects the quality and health of our water supply and the health of our waterways and oceans, including related wildlife—eventually affecting you and your family. And runoff can also cause erosion and structural problems to your property.

benefits

If you cut down your water usage, your pocketbook will benefit in many ways. By not overwatering you'll reduce the amount of replacement plants needed and urban runoff, while also protecting the look of your property. Furthermore, conserving water contributes to the reduction of public funds–intensive dam construction, which always has a negative environmental impact on the surrounding water, plant, and animal life. Reduction in watering and runoff also decreases the need for costly public storm-water processing, which helps prevent pesticides and pollutants from entering drinking water, rivers, and oceans. Less storm-water processing can either lower your local taxes or allow your city to allocate those funds elsewhere, where they could be put to better use.

how-to's

Fix Outdoor Water Leaks ☺ $

Check your outdoor hoses, pipes, and water taps for dripping water, and fix any leaks as soon as you can.

Water Your Lawn and Garden Early in the Morning ✚ ☺

Avoid evaporation of your irrigation by watering in the very early morning, not at night. If the plants and grass stay soaked for a long period of time (like overnight, if you water in the evening), fungus can begin to grow.

Check the Directions of Your Sprinklers ☺

There's no need to water your driveway, the sidewalk, or the side of your house! Not only is it a bad idea structurally, but you're also wasting money. Every few weeks, briefly turn on your sprinklers in the daytime to see if you need to replace a sprinkler head or adjust the direction a sprinkler is facing.

Install Drip Systems and Other Water-Efficient Sprinkler Devices ☺ $$-$$$

Drip systems emit small drops of water directly next to a bush or tree; this allows for specific and deep watering with a reduction in evaporation. Some cities and local hardware stores offer classes on how to install water-efficient sprinkler heads and drip systems, with many cities offering starter kits if you want to change to a drip system. Look for sprinkler heads and hose attachments that emit large drops instead of a fine spray, as the drops may reduce evaporation. Depending on your do-it-yourself expertise and your budget, you could also consider hiring a professional to help you redesign your landscape's irrigation system for more water efficiency.

RAINBIRD >> (www.rainbird.com) Another great company that has irrigation products such as timers, sprinklers, valves, and drip systems.

TORO >> (www.toro.com) This company offers high-quality irrigation timers, sprinklers, valves, and drip systems.

WATERSENSE >> (www.epa.gov/watersense) The EPA's WaterSense program is a great source for finding an experienced and certified irrigation specialist. There are certified WaterSense specialists in nearly every U.S. state.

Don't Hose Down Your Hardscapes ☺ ✿

Unless you need to reduce dust, avoid hosing down your hardscapes (driveway, sidewalks, steps); it simply wastes water and causes unwanted waste to be washed into the storm water system. If your sidewalk or driveway is dirty or covered with leaves, just sweep it. And use a rake instead of the hose to get rid of those leaves on the lawn. I cringe every time I see my neighbors hosing the leaves from their lawn and leaving them in a puddle of water for the city street sweeper to pick up. Talk about a waste of water and city resources! Those leaves could be put in the green waste recycling bin or saved for later use in a compost pile.

>> Don't let the hose run when you wash your car outside.

Install Water-Conserving Fountains ☺

If you want to install an ornamental fountain on your property, make sure it recycles its water. You'll just need to top off the water occasionally as it evaporates.

Grow Your Lawn to a Height of Three Inches or More ☺ ✿

Adjust your lawn mower to cut no lower than three inches. By growing a taller lawn, your grass's soil gets some shade, which reduces moisture evaporation and water needs—plus it helps prevent weeds. An easy way to determine your lawn's height is to step on the grass. If it bounces back, it isn't three inches long. If it lays flat, it's more than three inches.

Add Mulch to Your Garden ☺ ☼ $-$$

Adding mulch around your plants protects the soil from erosion and conserves moisture, which means you won't have to water as often. Mulch also keeps weeds at bay, which eliminates the need for herbicides, another environmental and health plus. Mulch is simply a protective layer of material that is spread over the soil. It isn't just wood chips! Mulch can be bought packaged from the hardware store or can simply be grass clippings from your last mowing. It also can be straw or matured material from your compost pile. (More about how to create and use a compost pile is found in chapter 4.) When I lived in Arizona, it was common for mulch to be small rocks that were spread all around the nongrass areas—the rocks didn't fertilize, but they did help to conserve moisture, prevent soil erosion, and reduce dust in the air. Any mulch should not be so compact that irrigation cannot reach the surrounding plants. *Consumer Reports* says that an ideal mulch depth to reduce evaporation is two to three inches.

Add Peat Moss to Your Yard and Garden ☺ $-$$

Adding peat moss to your soil helps it retain moisture, loosen and aerate, and retain nutrients. Your soil will soak up the moisture more readily and release it over a period of hours or days and will do the same thing with nutrients, which may mean you don't have to fertilize or add soil nutrients as often. Peat moss is environmentally friendly and doesn't have salts or chemicals in it, and it lasts several years with one application. You can put it on your lawn, in vegetable and flower gardens, and around trees and shrubs.

Buy and Use a Rain Barrel ☺ $$

Now, here's an innovative idea. If you place a rain barrel under your roof's rain gutter, you can catch rainwater and use it for your plants and garden. As a safety precaution, make sure the barrel has a secure top because you don't want children to be able to open up the barrel and get inside. Also, be sure it is on level, stable ground so that it won't tip over. Check the barrel regularly for overflow, and make sure it's empty in the winter (because it could form ice and expand, which would break the barrel).

Design a Xeriscape Landscape ☺ $$–$$$$

The word "xeriscape" (pronounced "zea-ree-scape") comes from the Greek word "xeros," which means "dry." A xeriscaped landscape plans for wise water use and conservation. The point of planting a xeriscape landscape is that you incorporate more native and drought-resistant greenscape into your property so that you can reduce your water usage and help the environment.

Native species are desired because not only do they survive better without extra maintenance, irrigation, and the reduced need for pesticides, but they also tend not to be invasive, meaning they will grow more in harmony with the surrounding environment instead of dominating and killing off other plants in their way (which can happen with nonnative species). Native species also support the surrounding ecosystem by offering the proper food, shelter, and nesting places for local and migrating birds. However, nonnative species, including invasive weeds, are a problem in many areas of the United States because they threaten the surrounding ecosystems, can degrade soil structure, and can cause more fire risks.

An easy way to build a xeriscaped garden or landscape is to add plant species that need infrequent-to-no artificial watering because they can survive on their own, as long as you have average rainfall. Some lawn grasses use more water than others, so if you're in an area that is dry, consider planting more hardy varieties, such as Bermuda. Consider ground covers and mulches, which can keep the soil moist longer and the weeds at bay. If you are watching your budget, swap out a tree here, a bush there, little by little, over time. You don't have to do it all at once.

a starter guide to xeriscaping

This basic table outlines several xeriscape starter plants, trees, and shrubs. For more ideas, check out your local Cooperative Extension System Office (more info in this chapter under Grow Healthy Produce, page 118), your state's department of water and conservation, or your local nursery. And most bookstores have gardening-specific books that focus on your particular region or climate. Additionally, the Natural Resources Conservation Service (www.nrcs.usda.gov) of the Department of Agriculture has a searchable database of thousands of plant species in the United States, including where they are considered native as well as other data and gardening information.

Region	Trees	Bushes	Other
Desert Southwest Climate: includes parts of Arizona, California, Nevada, New Mexico, and Southern Utah	Palo Verde Desert Willow California Fan Palm Arizona Mesquite Date Palm Silk Floss Tree Palo Brea Mulga Acacia Chinaberry	Bougainvillea Globe Mallow Ocotillo Bird of Paradise Lantana Sage (several varieties) Desert Honeysuckle	Desert Marigold (perennial flower) Verbena (groundcover) Barrel Cactus Century Plant Agave (succulent)
Mediterranean Climate/Coastal areas of California: includes Los Angeles and San Francisco	Arbutus Marina European Olive Crape Myrtle Black Acacia Pearl Acacia New Zealand Laurel Monterey Cypress Peppermint Willow	Abelia New Zealand Flax Escallonia Rockrose Rosemary Wild Lilac Lavender Bougainvillea Trumpet Vine	Deer Grass (decorative grass) Purple Fountain Grass (decorative grass) Society Garlic (perennial) Canyon Liveforever (succulent) Tapertip Liveforever (succulent)
Western Major Four-Season Climate*: includes the Inland Northwest, the West, and the less-arid portions of the Plains and Midwest	Rocky Mountain Juniper Piñon Pine Quaking Aspen (native to much of the United States) Desert Willow (drier areas of the West) Thinleaf Alder Mountain Mahogany Lodgepole Pine	Big Sagebrush Western Dogwood (limited Western United States) Broom Snakeweed Creeping Barberry Skunkbush Sumac	California Poppy (wildflower) Buffalo Grass (decorative grass) Snowball Sand Verbena (annual flower) Streambank Wild Hollyhock (subshrub)

*Cold winters, hot summers, wide temperature ranges in the fall and spring; lots of rain or snow in the winter with little to no rain in the summer. Requires hardy plants that can withstand extreme conditions.

Region	Trees	Bushes	Other
Temperate Rain Forest Climate: includes the coastal areas stretching from Northern California to Alaska	Pacific Dogwood Vine Maple Redwood (only in California and Oregon) Black Hawthorn (also grows along upper U.S. North 'from coast to coast) Beach Pine Sitka Spruce California Live Oak	Bog Rosemary Red Osier Dogwood (also good for much of the United States, except the South) Pacific Ninebark Salmonberry Salal California Wax Myrtle	Slough Sedge (grass) Lyngbye's Sedge (grass) Deer Fern Western Swordfern
Eastern Major Four-Season Climate**: includes the Great Lakes, New England, and some cooler areas of the lower Eastern United States	Staghorn Sumac Pitch Pine Northern Red Oak White Ash Eastern White Pine Sassafras Eastern Red Cedar	Lowbush Blueberry Pink Azalea Black Highbush Blueberry Wild Hydrangea Canadian Serviceberry	Canadian Wild Ginger (groundcover) Butterfly Milkweed (flowering plant, good for much of the United States except the Northwest) White Wood Aster (flowering plant) Spotted Geranium Virginia Bluebells (also native to the Southeastern United States)
Humid Subtropical Climate***: includes much of the Southeastern United States	Yellow Buckeye Carolina Hemlock Southern Sugar Maple Southern Arrowwood	Upland Swampprivet Carolina Buckthorn American Beautyberry	Pinkscale Blazing Star (perennial flowering plant) Wild Stonecrop (flowering ground cover)

* Although there are four distinct seasons, the seasons are more mild than northern areas of the United States.

*** Warm summer months and relatively mild winters with constant precipitation and humidity.

(continued)

Region	Trees	Bushes	Other
Humid Subtropical Climate *(continued)*	Needle Palm Southern Magnolia	Oakleaf Hydrangea Yaupon Roughleaf Dogwood (also tolerates colder temperatures in the Great Lakes area)	Pine Barren Deathcamas (perennial flowering plant) Virginia Spiderwort (flowering perennial)
Coastal Florida	Gumbo Limbo Scrub Hickory Button Mangrove Loquat (also native to Louisiana and California, produces fruit) White Stopper	Coco Plum Guianese Colicwood (small tree) Bahama Cassia Fiddlewood Yellow Necklace Pod	Aloe (also grows well in Texas and California) Iron Fern Cucumberleaf Sunflower (flowering groundcover) Seaside Goldenrod (native flowering perennial to entire Eastern U.S. seaboard)
Semi-Arid Climate in sections of the Great Plains****: includes parts of Texas, New Mexico, Nevada basin areas, and drier areas of Oregon and Washington	Saskatoon Serviceberry (also produces edible fruit) Utah Juniper Two Needle Piñon Rocky Mountain Ponderosa Pine Eastern Red Cedar (also native to Eastern United States) Gray Dogwood	Sand Sagebrush Big Sagebrush Four Wing Saltbush Mountain Ninebark Winterfat Soapweed Yucca	Prairie Sandreed (native grass) Western Wheatgrass (native grass) Buffalo Grass (native grass) Blue Grama (native grass) Leadplant (ornamental perennial) Big Bluestem (grass)

**** *Temperature ranges are extreme. Rainfall supports grasses but not forest cover.*

it's for the birds

Birds are able to tell us a lot about the health of our ecosystems—whether water supplies are contaminated; if there is enough natural habitat left for them to find sufficient food to eat, to find shelter, and to nest; or if there are toxic chemicals in their habitat. Unfortunately, common bird species are on the decline. According to the National Audubon Society's State of the Birds Web site (http://stateofthebirds.audubon .org), "since 1967 the average population of the common birds in steepest decline has fallen by 68 percent; some individual species nosedived as much as 80 percent."

The two most major threats to birds are loss of habitat and global warming.

Although the American Bird Conservancy and the National Audubon Society are involved in conservation efforts, you also have to do your part. One of the best things you can do is plant native plants and trees on your property. They provide the right kind of food, shelter, and nesting sites for birds that live and migrate in your area. Without these native plants and trees, the birds can't survive. You can also try xeriscape landscaping, discussed earlier in this chapter, which encourages native plant species.

Replace Your Real Lawn with Artificial Turf ☺ ✿ $$$–$$$$

We had a friend who hated to mow his grass. He dreamed of the day when he could purchase a synthetic lawn. That day finally came, and we were quite impressed. It looked and felt like real grass. No bugs, no mowing, no watering, no fertilizing, no expensive mowing or edging equipment, no gardener to pay, no grass pollen, no lawn mower pollution—it always looks green and is always the perfect length. If you do go this route, look for artificial turf that is made with recycled materials, and ask the company about recycling programs for your synthetic grass when it starts to fade and you want a replacement (within five to ten years).

Install a Weather-Tracking Watering System ☺ ✿ $$$–$$$$

If you have a large residential property, you can reduce your water usage by up to 60 percent and your runoff by up to 70 percent by installing an irrigation system that is only turned on when there isn't enough rainfall. You pay a company a service fee, and the system uses a special satellite to track humidity levels and rain patterns in your area. Some cities offer free systems or rebates for this type of watering program.

ETWATER >> (www.etwater.com) The company's smart-controller system uses weather data to automate and optimize your landscape watering schedules.

WEATHERTRAK >> (www.weathertrak.com) The company provides a weather-tracking irrigation service to help you save on water and improve the health of your plants.

eat, dress, spend green: be a conscious consumer

As a mom, you have a tremendous amount of buying power and influence. If your family is like mine, you are the one making the majority of decisions on what to buy, especially when it comes to everyday items like food, gardening supplies, household and personal care items, and clothes. Through your purchasing, you also shape what is produced and sold, because when a company sees there is an increased demand for a product or service, they will put more energy and supplies into it. The opposite is also true. As a result, when you make earth-friendly shopping choices, you shape what products are available to you. You can literally change the world by changing what and how you buy.

LIFESTYLE ACTION
think reduction

what you need to know

Let's just get it out in the open—we're all buying *a lot!* In today's world, people don't talk about keeping up with the Joneses anymore; most everyone is outbuying the Joneses. Maybe it's ubiquitous credit or the need to always have what's new. Peer pressure certainly contributes to the buying habit. When our buying is out-of-control, ironically we can also be left wanting more because today's purchasing habits are too often about using our money for the wrong things—stuff that is short-lived and decorative in nature, items that we impulsively pluck from the store shelves despite the fact that they contain little or no personal value.

Moreover, a lot of our purchasing over the last several decades has occurred without much thought about chemicals, waste, or how the product will affect us and our environment in the long run. But we now know that each of us is responsible for our health, our safety, and our environment. Therefore, a better future for your earth, your family, and your pocketbook is rooted in *reduction*—buying only what you need to be happy, safe, and healthy. This requires that you understand how your purchases affect your environment. Being a conscious consumer means you seek out practical ways to do more with less and you make purchases that are aligned with your values, which might include caring for your family, respecting nature and the environment, and embracing social responsibility. Bottom line—don't just buy something because of a cool ad or because your neighbors have it; a product has to offer real benefits and fall within your value system to be worth it.

> **THE CENTER FOR A NEW AMERICAN DREAM >>** (www.new dream.org) One of my favorite conscious-consumer organizations.

benefits
You can positively affect your bottom line and improve the health and safety of yourself, your family, and the environment by changing many of your shopping behaviors.

how-to's
Reduce How Much You Buy ☺ ✿
Before you pull out your wallet, consider if what you are buying is really *necessary*. While "necessary" is a subjective word, ask yourself if what you already have will do. Are you buying to satisfy a "craving" or to meet a need? Wanting and needing are two very different terms.

Dress and Decorate Eco-Smart +

As much as we all love them, fashion trends can quickly lead to more waste. Think of all the outfits we buy each season and discard once they're out of style. There is also widespread use of toxic chemicals to make and dye most clothes and textiles. Surprisingly, conventional cotton (a natural fiber), more so than polyester (man-made from petroleum), is one of the worse offenders in terms of of toxic chemicals and fiber dust being used in its production. Labor issues can also be a concern, as richer countries use poorer countries to make their fast fashion—a recipe for possible human rights abuses. Thankfully, we are more aware of these issues than ever before. As a consumer, you can help turn that awareness into a change. Here are some positive steps you can take:

> *Buy organic:* When you can afford to do so, buy clothing and textiles made from organic sources like organic cotton; this will help reduce the toxicity in the original fibers and its farming and make it a healthier product for you.

GLOBAL GIRLFRIEND >> (www.globalgirlfriend.com) Organic clothing and other eco-friendly and fair trade items.

THE GREEN LOOP >> (www.thegreenloop.com) Sells stylish eco-friendly clothing and accessories.

LOOMSTATE ORGANIC >> (www.loomstate.org) Organic cotton jeans.

NATURALLEE >> (www.naturallee.com) Fashionable sustainable furniture.

PATAGONIA >> (www.patagonia.com) Sells a number of durable organic and alternative fabric clothes, as well as clothes made from recycled polyester, and has a Common Threads Recycling Program.

(continued)

WHITE APRICOT >> (www.whiteapricot.com) Online newsletter and portal to fashion and beauty products that are ecologically and socially conscious.

Look for alternative fabrics: Hemp is one of the most interesting and diverse. It requires little-to-no pesticides or herbicides, less water to grow, and can be turned into more environmentally friendly silk, linen, knit, stretch, canvas, and muslin fabric blends. Ramie, flax, jute, sisal, coir, and bamboo are other alternative fabrics to keep an eye out for. Silk is another fabric that can be environmentally friendly. Lyocell (often heard of under its brand name of Tencel) is a new man-made fabric that is biodegradable, prevents bacterial growth, is chemical free, and is manufactured in a more environmentally friendly way—from cellulose found in wood pulp. There are also corn-based fabrics emerging, but if these fabrics are not organic and they cut into the food supply, they may not be your best choice. You can also look for recycled polyester fabrics.

BAMBOOSA >> (www.bamboosa.com) Sells bamboo clothing and accessories, and provides information about bamboo on its Web site.

HEMP TRADERS >> (www.hemptraders.com) Sells hemp fabric and provides lots of great information about hemp.

LENZING FIBERS >> (www.lenzing.com) Producers of Tencel, a Lyocell fabric—has more information about this fabric in the textile portion of the Web site.

Reduce the amount of clothing you buy: Stay current with today's fashions by adding a few new items or accessories, but try to avoid feeling like you have to change your whole wardrobe every season. Repair clothes instead of throwing them away—learn how to do some basic sewing so that you don't have to pay a tailor every time. This not only saves you money but also adds longevity to the clothes you have. When you are done with some clothing, don't throw it in the trash—donate it instead! Donated clothes will be worn by someone else or go to a recycling facility. Salvation Army (www.salvationarmyusa.org) and Goodwill (www.goodwill.org) are two great organizations to donate to.

Buy secondhand clothing: Save yourself money, help the environment, and be incredibly cool and hip by buying vintage and secondhand clothing. You can often make small alterations to used clothing for a newer look.

Lease or rent clothing: When you're using something short-term—wedding dresses, tuxes, maternity clothes, uniforms—consider leasing. A quick Internet search should lead you to places in your area.

Look for any eco-friendly labeling: There is no recognizable standard set yet for eco-friendly clothing, so be on the lookout for any emerging information from the manufacturer or brand that would state how the product was made (such as with less toxic dyes, less water, less energy, less pollution) and what it is made with (organic, biodegradable, renewable).

Look for Reusable ☺ ✿

We live in a disposable society that has a limited understanding of what it means to conserve. Companies sell us things that have a limited life—sometimes for convenience, but other times so that we'll buy more and pad their bottom lines. Unfortunately, our children are benefactors of multiple generations of overconsumption and nonreusability. I bet that if you take a hard look, you'll see yourself and your family underusing, overbuying, and overspending. To stop this expensive and wasteful cycle, you need to rewire your and your family's thinking. When you are shopping, think, "What can I buy that is reusable?" or "What might have a longer life span?" Here are some ideas:

Use reusable shopping bags: Bring along reusable shopping bags for groceries, mall shopping, or any kind of buying.

CHICOBAG >> (www.chicobag.com) Reusable shopping bags.

IKEA >> (www.ikea.com) Has reusable oversize totes for sale and encourages customers to not use plastic bags.

REUSABLE BAGS >> (www.reusablebags.com) Sells reusable shopping bags, reusable aluminum and stainless steel water bottles, and reusable lunch kits.

TARGET >> (www.target.com) This retailer sells a number of reusable shopping bags and totes.

>> Put your reusable bags in your car's trunk. That way you'll always have them with you when you go shopping.

Buy washable: If you have a choice between disposable and washable items, choose washable. Far too many disposable products take a long time to biodegrade; in the case of plastic, it's forever. Instead, reusable items allow you to conserve money and resources.

Avoid plastic water bottles: Nearly all plastic water bottles are made from oil, which means they are nonrenewable, non-biodegradable, and often pollute. Instead of petro-plastic water bottles, take water from the tap or filter your own water at home and then pour into an aluminum or stainless steel reusable water bottle, or if you're at home or at the office, use a washable cup or glass. By switching to a reusable water bottle or cup, a person can save $400–600 a year. Aluminum water bottles can be almost endlessly recycled, so they're a great choice for convenience. Another excellent alternative is bottled water that doesn't use oil for its packaging and instead uses plant material to make its plastic so that the plastic biodegrades and is compostable. This gives you the convenience without the guilt. And some traditional water bottle companies are also reducing the amount of plastic used in making their water bottles.

>> Look for shaving razors that let you replace the blade rather than use disposable razors. If you must choose disposables, recycle them. You may need to pop off the razor portion and recycle only the handle, depending on your recycling center's guidelines.

BRITA >> (www.brita.com) At-home water filtration by refrigerator filter, pitcher, or faucet mount.

NESTLE WATERS >> (www.nestle-watersna.com) This company has an Eco-Shape bottled water line under several brand names, which uses 30 percent less oil-based plastic than conventional plastic water bottles.

PRIMO >> (www.primowater.com) Bottled water that is in plastic bottles made from plants instead of oil. The bottles can be industrially composted. You can ask your local recycling center if they do industrial composting or you can find a list of industrial composting centers at Primo's Web site in the Frequently Asked Questions section.

PUR >> (www.purwaterfilter.com) Pitcher and faucet-mount at-home water filtration.

Choose rechargeable batteries: The estimated 15 billion single-use alkaline batteries produced and discarded each year pose a serious hazardous waste problem. Choose rechargeable batteries, and make sure used batteries get to your city's hazardous waste drop-off at the end of their life.

DURACELL >> (www.duracell.com) Has rechargeable batteries that can be charged hundreds of times.

ENERGIZER >> (www.energizer.com) Sells rechargeable batteries and chargers. Its NiMH (nickel-metal hydride) rechargeable batteries offer up to four times the performance when compared to old-technology rechargeables (nickel-cadmium batteries).

RADIO SHACK >> (www.radioshack.com) Sells a variety of rechargeable batteries and chargers.

Don't forget gently used options: Used clothing and furniture stores, including antique stores, offer an opportunity to get more use out of items that still have life. Or, consider joining a local online parenting group. Many of these groups share information not only about how to raise a family but also about clothing, toys, and furniture that members have available for sale or for free. Look for a group near you at www.groups.yahoo.com. Or you can check out a local Mothers & More chapter for in-person groups (www.mothersandmore.org).

Reduce plastic wrap and food storage bags: Put your food in reusable containers whenever possible. Make sure all plastic wrap and food storage bags are free of toxic chemicals like BPA and PVC, and plasticizers like DEHA and DEHP (all of which are described later in this chapter beginning on page 163).

GLAD >> (www.glad.com) Glad's food storage products are made from polyethylene (plastic #4) and polypropylene (plastic #5), and contain no PVC, BPA, plasticizers, or dioxins. And no dioxins are formed when heated. (More about dioxins can be found on page 163.)

SARAN >> (www.saranbrands.com) Plastic food wrap that is free of PVC and BPA. It is also dioxin free so that it can be heated safely in the microwave.

ZIPLOC >> (www.ziploc.com) Free of PVC, BPA, and dioxins, this company's plastic food bags and containers are also formulated not to contain harmful phthalates. The containers are plastic #5. The nonsteam and nonslider closure bags are plastic #4. Other bags with the slider closure and steaming capability are a mix of plastics 1, 4, and 5—and therefore would be considered a plastic #7 because of this mix. Plastic #7 is not toxic but is considered more difficult to recycle.

Consider reusable packaging for your move: Get used boxes from wine or liquor stores. The boxes with cardboard dividers make for easy packing of glasses and cups. Because they're made to transport full bottles, they're sturdy. Electronics retailers also have strong packaging, as their wares tend to be fragile. Boxes from the grocery store can also work, but they may retain smells or crumbs that can attract bugs. Read the outsides of the boxes for clues.

RENTACRATE >> (www.rentacrate.com) Reusable crates that you can rent, instead of using boxes, for your moving needs.

Reduce packaging: Always be diligent about refusing unnecessary packaging, and don't be afraid to speak up. If a clothing store wants to wrap your items in tissue paper, decline the tissue. If they put your clothing in a bag while it's still on a hanger, remove the hanger and leave it to be reused in the store. If you buy too many groceries and run out of reusable bags, request paper bags and discourage double bagging when it is not essential. Also, avoid buying products in single-serving packages. For example, buy a large jar of applesauce that can be portioned into reusable containers instead of single-serving applesauce portions (which create a lot more waste). Finally, some products, like electronics, are often unnecessarily overpackaged to create the illusion that there is more of the product inside than there really is. Make a better selection when you can, and if you must purchase something that is overpackaged, write the manufacturer to let them know you want that practice to change.

>> Another way to reduce packaging: Choose concentrated juice instead of fresh, because fresh is packaged in at least four times the amount of packaging. Fresh also costs more to deliver because of its water weight. If you really want fresh, liquefy fresh fruit in a blender or invest in a juicer—it will end up saving you money and time, as well as ensure up-to-the-minute freshness and quality.

>> When you can, choose paperless billing and ask to receive your statements by e-mail. You'll not only save time and postage, you'll save even more paper by not writing checks.

the diaper conundrum

Diapers are one of a new mom's biggest environmental hurdles. Your baby will use thousands of diapers before he or she is toilet trained. The vast majority of disposable diapers are made with plastic materials that do not biodegrade and are thrown into landfills. And many diapers are made with toxic chemicals. So, look for alternative choices:

Cloth diapers: Cloth diapering can save you more than half the cost of disposables. They are washable, available in organic cotton, and you can purchase flushable liners to help increase absorbency. Kushies (www.kushies.com) has fitted cloth diapers and both flushable and washable liners. gDiapers (www .gdiapers.com) have flushable and/or compostable inserts and a fitted cloth diaper.

Toxic-chemical free: Two great options are Tushies diapers at www.tushies.com or Seventh Generation (www.seventhgeneration .com).

And as for wipes, try using a warm wet washcloth like grandma did or use disposable wipes that have no fragrance, minimal chemicals (avoid chlorine), and are flushable/biodegradable.

Buy Local ✚ ☺

Buying local means looking for opportunities to purchase things, such as food, which were produced in or near your community. There may also be some money savings involved, as the manufacturer or supplier faces lower shipping costs to get the product to you. Shorter distance shipping also means less air pollution, and when food gets to you more quickly it will be fresher and last longer. Food items such as fruits and vegetables that are locally harvested offer added nutritional benefits because they were probably picked closer to being ripe and ready to eat. Buying local promotes community self-reliance, a diverse economy, and protects your food supply—all that is good for the environment and your pocketbook. There are three main ways you can support locally produced food:

Farmers' markets: Many communities have farmers' markets that sell locally produced food—primarily fruits, vegetables, honey, and eggs, as well as other items. Your local newspaper may list farmers' markets in your area. You can also check the U.S. Department of Agriculture's Agricultural Marketing Service's farmers' market search page at www.ams.usda.gov.

Community-supported agriculture: Also called CSA, this is an opportunity to regularly obtain locally produced food by subscribing to a farm's seasonal or regular offerings. Your membership with a farm grants you a share of their fresh crop, and many of these farms are organic. Each program is unique, but most entail picking up a box of food at a local pick-up point once a week or once a month; the box is typically a mix of whatever produce is in season. For poultry farms, you would get a delivery once every three months. Some CSAs also post seasonal recipes online. To find CSAs that deliver to your area, go to Local Harvest (www.localharvest.org).

Co-ops: A co-op is a special form of business or organization that is owned and run by a group of people who also use its services. A credit union is a good example. For food, there are co-op grocery stores in which the owners/members have a say in what is available for purchase and how the co-op is organized. Most co-op grocery stores are focused on local food, organic food, and vegetarian choices, and will sell to anyone, but its members usually receive a discount.

Ask your grocery store to stock local: Write a note to your grocery store requesting that locally grown food be purchased. Stores listen to people who take the time to voice their opinion and will often respond by fulfilling your request in order to gain your loyalty.

COOP DIRECTORY SERVICE >> (www.coopdirectory.org) An easy-to-use directory of co-ops is found on this site.

EAT LOCAL AMERICA >> (www.eatlocalamerica.coop) Information about local co-ops and farmers.

LOCAL HARVEST >> (www.localharvest.org) Excellent directory of farmers' markets, CSAs, local farms, and co-ops.

SLOW FOOD >> (www.slowfoodusa.org) A great organization that helps ensure your community has access to fresh and local food.

WAL-MART >> (www.walmart.com) Has a mandatory company policy of increasing its partnerships with local farmers. During the summer months, its grocery stores must purchase one-fifth of its produce from within each store's state.

WHOLE FOODS >> (www.wholefoods.com) Provides locally grown food at its stores.

stop the panic buying

Many moms think they don't have enough time to cook dinner, so all too often they end up getting pizza or fast food. Or, there are panicked end-of-the-workday runs to the grocery store, which frequently results in impulsive food buys for hungry tummies—with nutrition oftentimes going out the window. But it is healthier, better for the environment, and more cost-effective to make a homecooked meal. It works well if you plan ahead.

Stock up on healthy, easy-meal cookbooks: This way you'll have lots of ideas at your fingertips for making healthy food fast.

Stick to a shopping list: On the weekend, make a shopping list for the entire week. Use your cookbooks to come up with seven dinner entrees and write the necessary ingredients on your list. Add in produce, lunch and breakfast foods, and some stock-up items for your pantry and freezer so that your cupboards won't go bare so fast.

Buy everything for the week in one shopping trip: Just follow your list! This will save you time and gas money.

Consider cooking ahead: If you are really scrapped for time during the week, cook several entrees ahead of time on the weekend and either freeze or refrigerate for easy heat up. You'll also use less energy at home this way by heating the oven only once. Or, you can plan ahead and use a slow cooker. Put the ingredients in the cooker in the morning, and at the end of the day there is a warm homecooked meal waiting for you and your family.

Display produce in your kitchen: Stack up your fruits, squash, and melons in your kitchen. They will radiate beautiful color and also encourage your family to eat healthy snacks on the go. A diet laden with packaging-free produce is not only better for the environment but also better for your body.

Take a cooking class: If you don't know how to cook well, set aside some time to take a cooking class. Ask your kids to join you so that they can share in the responsibility of preparing family meals. This can save you time, and research shows that kids who get involved in making healthy meals are less overweight and more likely to be healthy as adults. The Association of Junior Leagues International (www.ajli.org) has a fun Kids in the Kitchen program that gets parents and kids involved in cooking healthy at home.

Gift Consciously ☺

Think eco-friendly, long lasting, and reusable when giving. Give gifts of time—like making someone a meal or cookies, teaching someone a new skill, going to the movies, going to the park—or gifts of health, like cooking classes or a gym membership. Or give gifts that last a long time—like living plants, timeless toys, or items made from things like sustainable bamboo or organic sources. Even giving to charities in someone's name as an alternative to buying a gift is a more conscious consumer way to go—an especially great idea for someone who has everything. For wrapping gifts, you can reuse materials such as newspaper, colorful pieced-together magazine pages, wallpaper scraps, and brown paper bags instead of traditional wrapping paper. You can also put gifts in reusable cloth bags or totes instead of buying throwaway gift bags.

> **BUY LESS CRAP >>** (www.buylesscrap.com) List of charitable causes you can donate to without buying, well, crap.
>
> **CHARITY NAVIGATOR >>** (www.charitynavigator.org) Lists and rates charities that you may be interested in giving to.
>
> **GREEN GIFT GUIDE >>** (www.greengiftguide.com) An online portal to sites that sell green products and gifts.

green party planner

If you're planning a party, it's a great opportunity to go eco! Send out electronic invitations instead of paper—www.evite.com is one option. If you must use paper, choose recycled whenever possible. Offer a buffet-style approach with more hors d'oeuvre-size portions so that people don't end up with as much waste on their plate. And either rent or borrow extra plates, utensils, cups, and napkins that are washable and reusable, or look for biodegradable or bamboo products. If you and your friends are unable to use leftover food, look into donating to a local food bank.

i'm dreaming of a green christmas

When it comes to Christmas trees, you may wonder what is the most eco-friendly tree choice—cut, live, or artifical? Live trees are a great choice if they'll be properly planted and taken care of once the holidays are over. Make sure they are of a variety appropriate for your region. Cut trees should be purchased from responsibly managed forests, then mulched afterward. A word of caution—while they can make your house smell great, they have a short life span and can bring air-polluting mold and bacteria into your home. Artificial trees have a much longer life span but should only be purchased if the manufacturer can certify the tree is not made with harmful chemicals or plastics (like PVC). Look for artificial trees that are made with nontoxic recycled materials and prestrung with energy-saving LED lights. Remember that after months of storage artificial trees can accumulate dust and mold spores. Be certain to air them out before bringing them indoors.

LIFESTYLE ACTION

consider what it's made of

what you need to know

I used to feel like I was the only person standing in the grocery store aisle reading a product's label, but recently I've noticed more and more fellow label readers. Knowing what goes into a product before you buy it is more important than ever. A product's labels can tell you the ingredients and/or materials; the nutritional value of foods; a product's origins; how to use and clean the product; hazards and safety precautions; risks and benefits; certifications and endorsements; the product's Web site; and other information. Additional facts and information, including the MSDS (which can further list ingredients and their potential hazards), can be found online.

As a conscious consumer, you need to carefully study what goes into a product before you buy it. Considering what a product is made of is important for the health and safety of your family because this information tells you how the product will eventually affect your environment. Also consider how much air pollution and energy was used to make and get the product to you, and if you should trust a brand because it was transparent and completely honest in distributing information.

benefits

The more you understand product labeling, the easier it will be for you to use this information to purchase healthier, safer, and more eco-friendly products. By being better informed, you may also save money.

how-to's

Stay Abreast of Product Issues ✚ ☺ $-$$

An informed and educated mom makes better decisions. One of the best ways to stay informed is by reading about current trends and issues. This can help you discern between marketing hype and the real truth. There are a number of periodicals and Web sites that can help you become an informed consumer. At my home, my regular consumer magazine subscriptions include the environment-focused *Plenty* magazine, the electronics and computer gadget monthly *PC World,* a subscription to the *Los Angeles Times,* and the magazines *Allure, Vogue,* and *Domino.* On an ad hoc basis, I'll read *Consumer Reports, Reader's Digest, Good Housekeeping, The Washington Post, National Geographic, Prevention, Glamour, O Magazine,* and daily news on Google.com. I also extensively search the Internet for credible information—often found on the Web sites of take-action and think-tank groups, many of which I list in the Resources section of this book, on page 289, and subscribe to a number of e-mail newsletters.

When I want to find out more about products and services directly from companies, I read up on their Web site—a company will usually talk about its environmental initiatives under topic areas like "green," "social responsibility," "environment," "investor," "about us," or under general company information. This is where you can learn about what they are disclosing in terms of their manufacturing processes and resulting products. Some forward-thinking companies will list how products are made on individual product Web pages or product categories. You want to patronize companies that are offering full disclosure and transparency of their operations, actual results (not just stating "we have a commitment to the environment" fluff), and a complete and documented environmental commitment from manufacturing to shipping. Here are key issues to search for:

- Are recycled components used in the manufacturing?
- Is the company making products that are recyclable or bio-degradable after use?
- Do the products have reusability and reduce waste?
- Have toxic and hazardous chemicals been reduced or eliminated?
- Is the company getting its ingredients or components from organic, sustainable, and renewable sources?
- Is the product's packaging more eco-friendly? Examples include using recycled materials, biodegradable packaging, and less packaging.
- Does the company eliminate water, air, and soil pollution from its manufacturing process?
- Is the company reducing its water and energy consumption?
- Does the company buy green energy or carbon offsets? (More about carbon offsets beginning on page 212.)
- Does the company have decentralized operations to keep manufacturing and shipping closer to the people who use the products? This is not always feasible, but localizing efforts can be more environmentally friendly and support local economies.

The point is that in today's world, there is no one-stop source for consumer information—it is found in many places and searching it out can take a good deal of work. The simple approach is to ask questions, then stick with brands you trust. Find a couple of magazines you think will inform you about the products you are buying, subscribe, and read them regularly. Subscribe to your local metropolitan newspaper or read it daily online—to save time, scan headlines for things that interest or affect you. And when you want to learn more about a particular subject, go Web surfing and do careful research; don't make a conclusion until you have found the same information from at least three credible sources.

what's fair is fair

The term "fair trade" is often tossed around next to other eco-friendly terms. True fair trade means that you are trading your money for something that was made under fair working conditions, purchased at a fair price (oftentimes directly from the producer instead of a middleman), and manufactured in a way that maintains a sustainable environment and helps to develop the community where it was purchased. One organization that provides a fair trade certification and related online directory is Transfair USA (www.transfairusa.org).

baby steps to being green

Alexandra Kennaugh created the Baby Steps initiative at the Natural Resources Defense Council's consumer Web site www.simplesteps.org. Being a new mom herself, she felt it was really important for mothers to realize what they need to do to protect their children—both short- and long-term lifestyle actions—and how to improve the health of the environment in which your child will grow up.

"I don't think being green is a fad," she says. "There are a great deal of people who are considering the environmental effects of their purchasing decisions. And moms will go green because it's so important for them and their young families and their posterity."

Alexandra feels that people need to be more active consumers. She encourages moms to ask about what is *not* on the label. "It is better to know more of the options and make the decision to go with more natural, more seasonal, and less of a carbon footprint—and it may not even cost you more," she says.

The idea of reducing your carbon footprint simply means that you're looking behind the kinds of products you're buying and asking questions such as:

- Did this product consume more energy or water than a competitor's? Examples of better choices include organic foods which consume less resources, concentrated products which use less water and cost less to transport, and companies that buy green power.

- Was the product shipped a greater distance than another option? You can often find this out by reading the label. Is it made in the United States or China? Will the product be shipped to you by air or ground? (Ground is less polluting.)

"If you like what a manufacturer is doing, write the company a letter and tell it what you liked so that the business knows where to put its attention," says Alexandra.

>> If you are going to shop online for a specific occasion—holidays or birthdays, for example—shop early. That way you'll have time to ship via ground (instead of air), which is a more eco-friendly and money-saving choice.

Read Labels ✚ ∅

Don't buy based on brand alone until you understand what goes into a brand's products. I know, for example, that if I buy products from Seventh Generation (www.seventhgeneration.com) or Aveda (www.aveda.com), I can trust the brand name alone. Both companies are making efforts to do right by me and by the environment. But the vast majority of products require you to do your homework and make your best judgment call, and carefully reading the label is the best way to know what you're buying—even if additional information is later found online. And while many ingredient lists read like a chemistry text, it is possible to educate yourself on what many of them mean. Food labels are the easiest to discern. The government's My Pyramid Web site (www.mypyramid.gov) teaches you a lot about food, and the U.S. Food and Drug Administration's Center for Food Safety and Applied Nutrition (www.cfsan.fda.gov) has lots of educational tools about how to read the nutrition facts label. You can read about cleaning ingredients in chapter 4.

Look for Its Origin ✚ ∅

Buy products made in the United States and, when necessary, from other countries that have similarly strict safety and health requirements. Additionally, when you buy close to home you are reducing the environmental impact of the product by not having to travel longer distances for it to reach your hands. To help you make more local choices, many products will list the city and state of the production facility or farm.

the truth about ranging and roaming
Understanding these terms will help you do your grocery shopping.

Free range, free roaming, cage free: Food labeled with one of these terms is supposed to mean that the animal has been allowed access to the outside. Unfortunately, even with this labeling, there have been widespread abuses by not allowing sufficient access outdoors. Not even "cage free" ensures sufficient access. Look for third-party certifications to verify the company's claims.

Grass fed, grain fed: Grass fed is an indication that the cow was pasture raised, though you need to read further; it is better if the label says "100 percent grass fed." Conversely, grain-fed cows would likely mean the animal did not have roaming access to pasture. Grain-fed poultry, however, is good because that means the poultry was fed grain over less nutritious and sometimes hazardous food, like bone meal.

Hormone free: This label is important on beef and means the animal was not treated with hormones. But it's already illegal to treat pork or poultry products, including eggs, with hormones.

Natural: This term may indicate that further details exist about eco-friendly, sustainable, or organic, nutritional value, or safety measures being taken, but there is no guarantee. And there are very few products that are actually regulated when using the term "natural" on their packaging. The few that are regulated are meats. Under the strictest USDA guidelines for meat and poultry, "natural" means that the product contains "no artificial ingredient or added color and is only minimally processed" and must explain what the term "natural" means on the package. For animal products, this label does not offer any indication of how the animal was raised.

Non-GMO: This means that the food has not been genetically modified. GMO stands for genetically modified organism. There is a worldwide movement against having foods genetically modified due to health and environmental concerns.

Pasture raised: Although the government does not regulate the use of this term, ideally this means that livestock lived in pastures where they could eat natural grasses and have fresh air and sunlight. Pasture-raised animals are humanely treated, healthier, and less susceptible to disease. This process also benefits the environment because manure acts as a natural fertilizer and less labor is needed to feed and maintain the animal. When it comes to human consumption, pasture-raised foods have been shown to have more vitamins and a healthier balance of fats.

rBGH free: This means that the animals were not given recombinant bovine growth hormones. The label is only allowed to appear on products from companies that have signed an FDA affidavit stating no hormones were injected in the animals. Other countries have gone beyond stopping rBGH voluntarily; both the European Union and Canada have banned rBGH in foods for human consumption.

NON-GMO PROJECT >> (www.nongmoproject.org) Information about genetically modified foods and an emerging non-GMO verification standard.

SUSTAINABLE TABLE >> (www.sustainabletable.org) This Web site helps to educate about problems with our current food supply and offers solutions and alternatives.

look for these two labels

A new label endorsed by the Humane Society and the American Society for the Prevention of Cruelty to Animals (ASPCA) is the Certified Humane label (www.certifiedhumane.com), which means the animal products (dairy, eggs, pork, lamb, poultry, and beef) you buy come from animals that ate a nutritious diet without antibiotics or hormones, and were "raised with shelter, resting areas, sufficient space, and the ability to engage in natural behaviors." For example, cows must have at least four hours of access to pasture or an exercise area each daily. These standards for animal welfare are more extensive than those required for organics, although you'll find products with both labels.

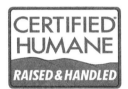

* Meets the Humane Farm Animal Care Program standards, Which include nutritious diet without antibiotics, or hormones, animals raised with shelter, resting areas, sufficient space and the ability to engage in natural behaviors.

Another emerging label is the Food Alliance Certified label (www .foodalliance.org), which is a nonprofit, third-party certification that means the farmer providing the food is engaging in sustainable agriculture, including both environmentally friendly and socially responsible production.

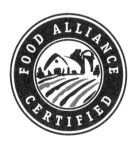

Recognize Third-Party Seals, Certifications, and Disclosures ✚ ⊘

These days many products have third-party endorsed seals, certifications, and disclosures that are imprinted on the label or found on a product's Web site. This information can be a quick reference for you to know that the product has passed some type of inspection and is expected to be safer, healthier, and more eco-friendly than other similar products without such an endorsement or disclosure. I have listed many seals, certifications, and disclosure information to look for throughout this book. If in doubt about a product's third-party certification or seal, you can always do an Internet search to see if it is authentic. Watch out for certifications that appear authentic but don't mean much—for example, there are some self-serving certifications that are actually created by the company itself with a phantom Web site in place to give the certifications credibility. And sometimes self-serving certifications are created by a consortium of companies solely to substantiate their own claims. Always check on the "about us" section of a certification's Web site to learn if the certifier is an independent (impartial) organization, the government, or sponsored by the product's company or companies. The sponsored-by entities are the questionable ones.

Stay Away from Toxic Products ✚

If you see the words "toxic," "dangerous," "caution," "warning," or anything remotely similar to those words on the product's label or in its literature, it should give you pause. MSDSs are available either online or on the label or packaging for some products, and these sheets should give a full, unbiased disclosure of ingredients and indicate hazardous components. Here's a simple rundown of what to avoid:

Any product labeled with "chlorine" or "chlorine-processed." Instead, choose products labeled "chlorine free." Chlorine-free paper and cleaning supplies are good examples.

Traditional pesticides, herbicides, and fertilizers. Instead, choose organic or other alternatives like using compost. I give lots of ideas in chapter 5.

Mercury. Much of today's common lighting contains mercury; it is unavoidable and simply needs to be disposed of as hazardous waste; more about lighting is found in chapter 2. Lots of fish are also known to have high mercury levels and should be avoided—see page 175 for more information.

>> Buy only digital thermostats and thermometers and avoid those made with mercury.

>> If you do crafts that require painting, make sure the paint pigments do not contain mercury.

>> At your next dental visit, ask to have your old mercury fillings replaced with composite, porcelain, or resin.

Lead. Look for lead-free toys and dinnerware. Lead-free can only be determined by the manufacturer stating the product is lead-free. If a product says "Made in the USA," there is a good chance the product is lead-free as long as any imported parts were also lead-free.

BEYOND LEARNING >> (www.beyond-learning.com) Kids' learning games printed with soy ink on recycled paper.

PLANTOYS >> (www.plantoys.com) Environmentally friendly toys.

PVC. All plastic labeled #3 is made using polyvinyl chloride (PVC). PVC and the other chemicals used to make it release poisonous chemicals throughout its lifetime, including mercury, dioxins (toxic compounds known to increase your cancer risk), chlorine, lead, and phthalates (makes hard plastics soft and has multiple harmful health effects). PVC products are everywhere, including vinyl shower curtains, children's and baby's toys, plastic wrap, most artificial Christmas trees, electronics, food containers, building materials (windows, doors, piping, fixtures), and beverage bottles. If you see the number 3 or letter "V" under the universal recycling symbol on any product, avoid purchasing it, and choose an alternative. If you already own any #3 plastic food containers, recycle them or use them for nonfood items like organizing nails in the garage. If you're not sure what type of plastic is being used on your children's or babies' toys, pacifiers, or teething rings, throw them in the recycling bin and look for alternatives. And ask electronics manufacturers if PVC is used in their products. (See an informational table on plastics and their labeling in chapter 4.)

BPA. Plastic #7 is often made of polycarbonate plastic, which is made from a chemical called Bisphenol A (BPA). BPA is a health hazard, interfering with reproductive development and hormones. Avoid purchasing #7 plastic for any food or beverage use because BPA can leach into foods. BPA is also currently used to line the inside of most metal food and soda cans, so drink less canned soda and eat less canned food whenever possible, and write your state and federal representatives to ask for BPA-free legislation. Environmental Working Group (www.ewg.org) performed independent testing in March 2007 and found unsafe levels of BPA in one of every ten servings of canned foods (11 percent) and one of every three cans of infant formula (33 percent). Avoid baby bottles or sippy cups made from polycarbonate #7 plastic because BPA can leach into your baby's formula or drink. Plastic bottle liners are also dubious. Instead, choose glass or polypropylene #5 plastic because neither have BPA, and choose silicone nipples. Environmental Working Group recommends powdered formula in safe plastic containers.

>> Safer plastic food containers will be labeled 1, 2, 4, or 5. Or choose metal (BPA-free aluminum or stainless steel) or glass.

BORN FREE >> (www.newbornfree.com) Nontoxic baby bottles, nipples, and drinking cups.

GREEN TO GROW >> (www.greentogrow.com) Baby bottles free of phthalates and BPA, and silicone nipples.

NURTUREPURE >> (www.nurturepure.com) Sells toxin-free glass baby bottles, and silicone, chemical-free nipples.

Phthalates and plasticizers. These are chemicals that soften or make various consumer products more flexible, including electronics; and are often added to PVC to make it softer and pliable. Phthalates are also added to cosmetics and personal care products to carry fragrances. However, phthalates and plasticizers have detrimental health effects and should be avoided whenever possible. By avoiding PVC products, you will eliminate a good deal of phthalates and plasticizers from your life. Some of the more common phthalates are DEHP, BzBP, DEHA, DBP, DEP, and DMP. If in doubt, you can ask a manufacturer if any plasticizers or phthalates were used to make a product.

Flame retardants. Many electronics, furniture, and plastics manufacturers use flame retardants in their products, and many flame retardants are industrial toxic chemicals. They are known as brominated flame retardants (BFRs) or polybrominated diphenyl ethers (PBDEs). These flame retardants not only migrate from products, often as dust, and build up in the bodies of animals and humans, but they also pollute the water because they do not degrade. Additionally, when items with flame retardants are recycled, the toxic chemicals are released into the air. Buy products that are BFR- and/or PBDE-free whenever possible. The EPA's DfE program (www.epa.gov/dfe) is also partnering with companies and organizations to find alternatives to traditional flame retardants.

PFCs. Currently most stain- and stick-resistant products, such as pans treated with nonstick substances or sofas sprayed with stain-resistant chemicals, have what are called perfluorinated compounds (PFCs). The chemicals used to make PFCs—PFOA (perfluorooctanoic acid) and PFOS (perfluorooctane sulfonate)— are getting attention as health and environmental hazards. Products that may contain PFCs include grease-resistant packaging (like microwave popcorn bags), carpets, furniture, water-resistant clothing, nonstick cookware, dental floss, and much more. Read labels or call manufacturers to determine if they have eliminated or reduced their use of PFCs. And for cookware, look for PFC-free cast-iron options such as pots made by Le Creuset (www.lecreuset.com) or Lodge (www.lodgemfg.com).

VOCs. Volatile organic compounds are toxic and pollute the air you breathe. They are found in alcohol, methanol, isopropanol, mineral spirits, glycol ethers, formaldehyde, and strong plant oils (terpenes). Strong-smelling products may contain VOCs. Look for products that overtly state they have low or no VOCs.

Other toxic chemicals. Avoid products that contain lye, hydrochloric acid, phosphoric acid, sulfuric acid, ammonia and ammonium compounds, phosphates, EDTA, petroleum, diethylene glycol, nonylphenol ethoxylate, butyl cellosolve, monoethanolamine (MEA), alkylphenol ethoxylates (APEs), paraffin, mineral oil, perchloroethylene, and antibacterial agents like triclosan and benzalkonium chloride. See chapter 4 for more information on these and other chemicals.

CENTER FOR HEALTH, ENVIRONMENT & JUSTICE >>
(www.chej.org) Has helpful campaigns and information that can
help protect you and your family from exposure to dangerous environmental chemicals.

CONSUMER PRODUCT SAFETY COMMISSION >> (www.cpsc
.gov) U.S. agency that is responsible for protecting consumers
from serious injury or death from more than 15,000 types of products; lists recalls and product safety news on its Web site.

COSMETIC SAFETY DATABASE >> (www.cosmeticsdatabase
.com) Type cosmetics by name into the search engine and learn
about any chemical hazards. This Web site also has a parent's buying guide for children's personal care products.

GREENPEACE >> (www.greenpeace.org) Has a very helpful annual online guide to greener electronics that easily breaks down
how some of the biggest companies are doing when it comes to
toxic chemical elimination and recycling programs.

**NATIONAL INSTITUTES OF HEALTH'S HOUSEHOLD PROD-
UCTS DATABASE >>** (http://householdproducts.nlm.nih.gov)
Online database of household products, their ingredients, and their
MSDSs.

POLLUTION IN PEOPLE >> (www.pollutioninpeople.org) Information on toxic chemicals and their safer alternatives.

SIGG >> (www.mysigg.com) Sells high-quality, non leaching aluminum bottles and containers that also are fashionable—the aluminum is also completely recyclable.

(continued)

SILICON VALLEY TOXICS COALITION >> (www.etoxics.org) Has lots of great information on choosing high-tech products that are safer. Publishes purchasing guides for more environmentally friendly and less toxic electronics.

THERMOS >> (www.thermos.com) Sells BPA-free, nontoxic beverage bottles made of stainless steel.

WASHINGTON TOXICS COALITION >> (www.watoxics.org) Education and advocacy group for safer products, including lead-free toys.

look for the leaping bunny

Many cosmetics and personal care items are labeled "cruelty free" or "not tested on animals" but there is not a third-party certification that verifies that what the company is stating is actually true. Also, there is a loophole—the raw materials might have been tested on animals, but the final product was not. In any case, it is always better to look for reliable, third-party verification of any claims. One such certification you can look for is the Leaping Bunny (www.leapingbunny.org), which means "no new animal testing is used in any phase of product development by the company, its laboratories, or suppliers."

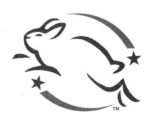

>> Look for palm oil–free products. Palm oil and palm kernel oil are used as a common additive in soap, cosmetics, and food

products, and come to us at the expense of destroying rain forests by fire—mostly in Indonesia and Malaysia, where 25,000 square miles have been ruined—to clear the way for more palm oil plantations. These destroyed habitats adversely affect endangered wildlife like tigers and orangutans, not to mention the extensive carbon dioxide released into the air from burning. Instead, you can choose products with canola or olive oil. Write your government representatives to ask for a ban on palm oil.

AVEDA >> (www.aveda.com) The company and its personal care products are dedicated to product safety, responsible ingredient sourcing, utilizing more natural and organic ingredients, reducing packaging *and* using recycled materials in its packaging, and powering its operations with renewable energy.

THE BODY SHOP >> (www.thebodyshop.com) The company has a strict policy against animal testing its ingredients and products. It also supports fair trade.

GREEN BY NATURE >> (www.greenbynaturebeauty.com) Personal care products that are 100 percent paraben, DEA, and sulfate free.

ORIGINS >> (www.originsorganics.com) The company has a USDA Organic–certified line of skin, body, and hair care products.

PHYSICIANS FORMULA >> (www.organicwearmakeup.com) Sells an Organic Wear line of cosmetics that is 100 percent free of harsh chemicals and synthetic preservatives and colors, 100 percent cruelty free, 100 percent free of parabens and GMOs,

(continued)

uses up to 93 percent less plastic for some of its containers, and integrates U.S.-certified organic ingredients into this product's line.

burt's bees began with a mom who cared

The popular natural beauty company Burt's Bees (www.burtsbees.com) began with a beekeeper named Burt and a mother of twins, named Roxanne Quimby, who wasn't in the best of financial situations. In 1984, Roxanne came up with a business plan and started making beeswax products with Burt. Since then, she has become an advocate for conserving Maine's land and wildlife, and she has not backed down from sticking to using renewable resources, a safe cosmetics policy, and nearly 100 percent natural ingredients.

Buy Organic ✚

I cannot stress enough the importance of buying organic. When a food, animal, or material is certified organic, that means that you:

- Don't have to worry about toxic chemicals—organics are grown without any synthetic chemicals (no synthetic fertilizers, pesticides, or herbicides); this protects your family's health and the land's well-being; and nearly eliminates toxic runoff which alters and kills life in waterways and oceans.
- Don't have to be concerned about irradiation, genetic modifications, antibiotics, or hormones—organic food has been produced with none of the above.
- Support food that is grown in better and healthier soil, which leaches less nitrogen, holds more nutrients (which can be passed onto your food and ingredients), and produces less runoff and erosion.
- Support food security. When buying organic food, you are securing the health of the soil and conserving water. Yet the

same or more food is produced off the same acre of land compared to conventionally grown food.

- Support a healthy pollinator and bird population. Bees and other pollinating insects, as well as birds, are killed and adversely affected by toxic chemicals.
- Support outdoor access for animals and pasture access for livestock.
- Support animals eating 100 percent organic feed.

Everything listed above benefits you and your family's health and the sustainability and health of the planet. While organic options are available in many places, the more people buy it and demand it from their stores, the more available it will become and, as a result, prices will decrease. If you can't afford to buy all organic foods, concentrate on buying a few organic items such as baby food, or organic produce that would otherwise have the highest pesticide residue—apples, grapes, green peppers, peaches, and pears. This gives the most bang for your organic buck.

Be sure to look for the USDA Organic label. It can *only* be used on products that are at least 95 percent organic.

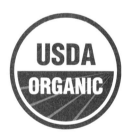

If you see other products with the words "organic" but no USDA Organic label, read the label carefully for other details. The USDA allows processed products with at least 70 percent organic ingredients to use the phrase "made with organic ingredients" but the USDA Organic seal cannot be used anywhere on the package. If a product has less than 70 percent organic ingredients, then according to the USDA the word "organic" cannot be used anywhere on the packaging except for listing organic items in the ingredients list. You should report products that misuse the word "organic" to the USDA.

food safety stays tops

Whether you buy organic produce or not, make sure your food is properly cleaned to reduce the chance of you ingesting any bacteria, dirt, or chemicals (for nonorganic). Do not soak produce; rather, rinse it under running tap water for at least several seconds. Firm-skinned fruits and vegetables can also be rubbed with your hands or scrubbed with a vegetable brush under running water. Do not use bleach or detergent to wash produce, as you could make yourself sick with any consumed residue.

rethinking flowers

When buying cut flowers, look for the USDA Organic seal, as nonorganic flowers can be just as polluting as nonorganic food. Try to buy your flowers locally and in season whenever possible, because shipping flowers for next-day delivery via air is highly polluting. The Association of Specialty Cut Flower Growers (www.ascfg.org) has an online, state-by-state buyers' guide that you can search. And Local Harvest (www.localharvest .org) has info on nearby farms. You can also look for Veriflora-certified flowers (www.veriflora.com), which means that the flowers have been grown and sold in a sustainable way (environmentally, socially, and economically).

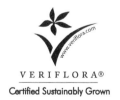

VERIFLORA®
Certified Sustainably Grown

CALIFORNIA ORGANIC FLOWERS >> (www.californiaorganic flowers.com) USDA Organic flowers.

THE CORNUCOPIA INSTITUTE >> (www.cornucopia.org) Has a helpful online dairy report and scorecard to determine the integrity of your organic milk.

DIAMOND ORGANICS >> (www.diamondorganics.com) Sells a wide variety of organic foods and flowers.

ENVIRONMENTAL WORKING GROUP >> (www.foodnews.org) This Web site has a Pesticides in Produce guide.

NATIONAL ORGANIC PROGRAM >> (www.ams.usda.gov/NOP) This is the USDA's site for information on and regulation of the USDA Organic label. There is also information on how to file a complaint.

ORGANIC BOUQUET >> (www.organicbouquet.com) Organic flowers and gifts.

ORGANIC CONSUMERS ASSOCIATION >> (www.organic consumers.org) Excellent source of information and public issues awareness about organic products.

ORGANIC VALLEY FARMS >> (www.organicvalley.coop) A nationally distributed farmer-owned co-op of organically produced dairy and other farm products, including milk, cheese, butter, eggs, orange juice, soy beverages, produce, and meats.

TRADER JOE'S >> (www.traderjoes.com) Grocery store with excellent selection of organic food products. It also has one of the best budget-friendly selections of organic and cage-free eggs.

WHOLE FOODS >> (www.wholefoodsmarket.com) Large variety of organic products; also has a number of programs in place to support local growers.

Eat Less Meat ✚ ☺

Eating a diet richer in plants than in meat not only benefits your health but also helps the planet. For your health, a more plant-based diet means less chronic disease and less foodborne illness. For the planet and your overall environment, less of a demand for meat means less will be produced, which in turn helps to cut down on the amount of manure and noxious gases that need to be properly disposed of. Yes, gases. You see, livestock produce about one-fifth of the world's greenhouse gases due to, well, their own gas—which includes methane—and waste (manure has lots of ammonia). In fact, the United Nations considers livestock one of the world's most serious environmental problems and has reported that cattle rearing across the world contributes more greenhouse gases into the atmosphere than driving vehicles does. Part of the problem, say some researchers, is that there are too many cows that are overfed grain, which causes more gas and chemicals to gather, instead of being reared on grass and pastures.

Another problem is the world consumption of beef is increasing as many societies that once ate little to no meat are westernizing. The result is a rising global demand for livestock, which leads to the clearing of forests so there's a place to put the cows, which, in turn, leads to animal gas and waste, plus production and distribution of the meat—all of which contributes to pollution.

Many would argue, then, that everyone should become vegetarian or vegan, but I am not recommending that. If you want to, great. But what everyone can do is simply to cut down on meat consumption. It's best for the planet and your body. An easy way to do this is to eat only one burger a week instead of two. Learn how to make a balanced meal with beans, legumes, tofu, or edamame instead of meat. Or add two vegetable and fruit sides to your meal, instead of one, to fill you up.

As long as you understand how to get the right nutrients from a variety of foods, the health benefits are numerous. A diet lower in meat can reduce your risks of heart disease and cancer. Finally, you can also save money. By reducing how much meat you buy and instead substituting with such things as beans, lentils, nuts, seeds, tofu, and soybeans, you can easily cut your main protein costs by two thirds. That money saved can be either pocketed, used to buy more veggie and fruit options, or used to buy more organic produce without going over your food budget.

renewable versus responsible

"Renewable" is a word that is frequently tossed around to connote environmentally friendly. But unfortunately renewable doesn't always mean responsible. Renewable means that a source material that a product is made from can be renewed and not depleted. For example, corn products are considered renewable because you can re-plant corn again and again, whereas petroleum is not considered renewable because once you've pumped out the last drop, that's all there is.

However, the big problem with simply stating "renewable" is that it tells you nothing about how the growing, harvesting, production, or manufacturing was conducted. For that, you need more information. For example, one of the most troubling problems with products made with corn is that while corn is renewable, it is often not farmed responsibly. It is rarely grown organically, lots of toxic chemicals (pesticides, herbicides, fertilizers) are used, and there are problems in managing how much corn is being raised for human and animal consumption versus emerging bioproducts like alternative fuel. The bottom line in all this is that you want to purchase not only renewable but also responsible products. The only way to do this is through research, asking questions, and reading labels.

Stick with Sustainable and Safe Seafood ✚

Seafood is healthy, right? Well, you'll be surprised to know that much of the fish you've grown up eating and fed your children, especially tuna, is probably not all that healthy. For decades we've polluted our oceans with toxic waste and trash. Metals such as mercury and lead, pesticides, and industrial chemicals such as PCBs (polychlorinated biphenyls) have accumulated in the marine environment and its fish. Once you eat those fish, the same contaminants accumulate in your body and can cause developmental problems, create a cancer risk, and bring about mercury poisoning. Additionally, overfishing and abusive fishing is a tremendous problem that is killing off whole groups in marine ecosystems.

One such example is in the shrimp industry, in which widespread labor and ecological abuses abound, including the destruction of mangroves (forests in coastal waters) that are vital to sea life, help stem erosion, and protect the coast from storms. When you buy cheap shrimp, you are contributing to these abuses and problems.

Finally, global warming is heating ocean waters and destroying habitats. As a result, if these current trends continue, credible reports say that the ocean's ecosystems are expected to collapse in the next forty years. This is an urgent call to action for moms, families, and businesses everywhere! Only buy seafood that is considered sustainable and safe. Insist on fish that has been responsibly managed and fished, and therefore likely to be less contaminated. And you should know that currently there is no standard for organic seafood, so any brand that makes that claim better have documentation to back up its statements.

ENVIRONMENTAL DEFENSE FUND >> (www.edf.org) Has lots of well-documented information about seafood and contaminants, including a helpful rating of fish oil supplements.

GOT MERCURY? >> (www.gotmercury.org) Has an online mercury calculator to help you determine how to make healthier seafood choices.

MANGROVE ACTION PROJECT >> (www.mangroveactionproject .org) Action group that encourages protection and better management of coastal environments and tackles abuses in the shrimp industry.

SEAFOOD WATCH >> (www.seafoodwatch.com) The best responsible-shopping-for-seafood help that I have found is through

California's Monterey Bay Aquarium's program called Seafood Watch. Every year the organization offers online guides that you can print out and take with you when you go shopping or eat out at a restaurant.

>> The blue Marine Stewardship Council label (www.msc.org) is found on fish products that come from certified fisheries that do not overfish, have minimal impact on the marine environment, and are able to remain sustainable from season to season.

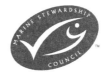

speak up if you want to be heard

One of the best ways to insure that you will have more environmentally friendly, healthier, and safer products to buy is by letting manufacturers know that that is what you want. Although I discuss expressing your opinion in more depth in chapter 9, I'll reiterate the fact that your voice is important. Companies know that if one person took the time to articulate a belief, thought, or concern, then there are hundreds if not thousands of other such people who did not take the time to do so—but feel just the same way. Your comments are taken seriously by companies as a representative sample of their customers and can make serious changes in manufacturing, product sourcing, and ultimately, the item you have to buy.

Not too long ago I was frustrated with not being able to find cage-free and organic eggs in my local supermarket. So I went home, typed up a request in the suggestion area of the supermarket chain's Web site, and by that evening had a personal response. Within a week, and ever since, there are abundant cage-free choices at my store. That was from one person's voice. Here are ways you can easily express an opinion:

Go online. Nearly all companies have a way to contact them and give feedback online.

Call the customer service line. This is another easy way to express your opinion.

Write a letter. A carefully thought-out letter directed to the president of the company (and I don't care if it's the president of Ford Motors!) will get their attention.

Suggestion card. Ask the store if they have a suggestion card when you check out; these cards will often have postage already paid for you.

Reduce Your Need for Pharmaceuticals ✚ ☺

By no means should you reduce or eliminate your prescription and any necessary over-the-counter (OTC) medications without consulting with your physician, but look for ways to prevent the need for those conventional medications. Not only can your health improve, but there are also tremendous gains for the entire environment and how it affects you in the long-term.

Prescription and OTC meds are considered hazardous waste and their use has been steadily rising. From 2002 to 2007 prescription drug use rose by 12 percent. And unfortunately, the medicinal waste that flows through our sewers is often not able to be fully treated in water-treatment plants, so residue flows back into lakes, streams, and the ocean. The result is a contamination of our water supply and a radical effect on marine and water life.

In a five-month investigation by the Associated Press in 2008, drugs were detected in the drinking water supplies of twenty-four major metropolitan areas. The drugs discovered included micro doses of such meds as antibiotics, anticonvulsants, mood stabilizers, sex hormones, ibuprofen, acetaminophen, and heart-problem medication. In the same AP report it was found that in Philadelphia alone, there were fifty-six pharmaceuticals or medicinal-type by-products found in treated drinking water. To make matters worse, our federal government has no requirements for any drug-residue testing of drinking water—an obvious loophole in the system. Additionally, the toxic soup created by these pharmaceuticals and other hazardous waste dumping in waterways, lakes, and the ocean has resulted in altering the hormone structures and overall health of marine life—feminizing male fish, impairing reproduction, depressing wildlife immune systems and organ functions, and causing deformities.

In addition to reducing your need for medications, ask questions about what is in the medicine, of any kind, that you are taking, and ask your municipality's waste-treatment plant what they are doing to reduce any medicinal waste residue from wastewater. Look into alternative medicine options that can help you get to the root cause of a chronic or acute health problem, again helping you to eventually avoid conventional medications, which sometimes mask symptoms of a greater problem. Some excellent prevention-based treatments are homeopathy, naturopathy, acupuncture, and chiropractic.

THE AMERICAN ASSOCIATION OF NATUROPATHIC PHYSICIANS >> (www.naturopathic.org) Has a searchable ND database on its Web site.

AMERICAN CHIROPRACTIC ASSOCIATION >> (www.amerchiro.org) Has chiropractic information and an online chiropractor search feature.

THE COUNCIL FOR HOMEOPATHIC CERTIFICATION >> (www.homeopathicdirectory.com) Lists a directory of certified homeopathic professionals.

(continued)

NATIONAL CENTER FOR COMPLEMENTARY AND ALTERNA-TIVE MEDICINE >> (www.nccam.nih.gov) A good U.S. government reference site for emerging information on preventive and complementary care.

NATIONAL CENTER FOR HOMEOPATHY >> (www.national centerforhomeopathy.org) Has study groups across the United States to learn more about homeopathy.

NATIONAL CERTIFICATION COMMISSION FOR ACUPUNC-TURE AND ORIENTAL MEDICINE >> (www.nccaom.org) Has information on acupuncture and oriental medicine.

green on the go:
move and play green

Think about how much time you spend traveling, and I don't just mean your annual family vacations. There's heading to work, running around town shopping, taking the kids to soccer practice, and enjoying everyday recreation. No matter where your travels take you, you can be greener—to benefit your pocketbook, your health and safety, and your environment. And while there are always new advances in technology to help you do this, a good majority of going green for travel and recreation comes with your choices and behaviors—all of which can be integrated into your overall wellness lifestyle.

LIFESTYLE ACTION

use alternative transportation whenever possible

what you need to know

When I'm driving around town to pick up my kids from school, get the dry cleaning, hit the gym, or buy groceries before dinnertime, I'm a woman on a mission, and find it hard to think about anything else other than where I need to go and what I need to get. I do, however, try to remind myself that every trip in the car has a negative effect on my environment. The reality is that, according to the EPA, *one third* of the air pollution in the United States is caused by tailpipe emissions from cars and trucks—

including my car. Vehicles mainly emit four types of significant air pollutants:

Carbon monoxide is an invisible, poisonous gas that can neither
be seen nor smelled. It reduces the amount of oxygen delivered
to your body and its tissues and can also irritate your lungs and
give you a headache. Over 50 percent of carbon monoxide
gases come from vehicles of all kinds; in some cities it can be as
high as 95 percent.

Hydrocarbon and nitrogen oxide are irritating pollutants to the
lungs and the heart and can also be toxic and cancer-causing.
When you combine hydrocarbons and nitrogen oxide (also called
nitrous oxide) with sunlight, you get what is called ground-level
ozone—one of the main components of smog. The more sunlight,
the more ground-level ozone is produced (that's why summer
smog is worse). Plus, ground-level ozone can be transported by
the wind to other areas hundreds of miles away—so what
happens in your town affects others as well.

Particulate matter is emitted from all types of vehicles, but
especially those that are diesel powered. It's comprised of little
bits of particles that can float in the air for as much as a third of a
mile from the original emission, be inhaled, and lodge themselves
in the deepest parts of your lungs, leading to breathing problems
such as asthma and chronic bronchitis. And the Natural
Resources Defense Council says that 64,000 people die each
year because of particulate air pollution—compare that to
418,000 people dying each year from smoking-related causes.

Greenhouse gases contribute to global warming (the trapping of
too much heat in the earth's atmosphere). Fuel burning from
vehicles releases carbon dioxide (CO_2) into the atmosphere.

In addition to these air pollutants, vehicles also release air toxins,
which have been proven to be cancer-causing. Because all these

emissions occur when you use traditional—and even many hybrid—forms of transportation, whenever possible look for alternative modes of transportation that can eliminate or reduce emissions.

benefits
You can help to protect the health and safety of your family and immediately improve your environment by choosing alternative modes of transportation.

the good, the bad, and the ozone
Ozone is a gas that can be good or bad for your health and the environment, depending on its location in the atmosphere.

Bad ozone, also called ground-level ozone, is essentially what we know as smog. It's bad for your health (it can cause chest pain, coughing, throat and lung irritation, congestion, and much more) and it damages crops, trees, and other vegetation. Bad ozone is created by chemical reactions in the emissions from factories and electric utility companies, motor vehicle exhaust, gasoline vapors, and chemical solvents. Heat makes bad ozone worse, almost like a cooking effect, which is why summer smog is so dangerous. This type of ozone can be reduced by:

- Conserving energy
- Reducing vehicle use
- Using less gas-powered equipment
- Avoiding products with high VOCs, such as many paints and finishes, cigarettes, carpets, cleaning products, and some furnishings

Good ozone is what cocoons the earth, protecting it from getting too much of the sun's harmful UV rays. Good ozone is high up in the atmosphere—it starts about six to ten miles above ground and goes up to about thirty miles above the earth. It's important to maintain this good ozone layer for everyone's protection, but unfortunately, over the years, it has been depleted by products that emit substances like chlorofluorocarbons (CFCs) and hydrochlorofluorocarbons (HCFCs). CFCs and HCFCs were once commonly found in coolants, fire extinguishers, solvents, aerosols, and pesticides. When you hear "there's a hole in the ozone," they are talking about documented satellite measurements of the thinning of this protective ozone layer, particularly over the polar regions. With this good ozone thinned out, we get more UV radiation, which can lead to more cases of skin cancer, damage to crops, and warming of the polar regions and oceans, killing off important pieces of that food chain.

how-to's

Walk ☺ ✚

Put on those walking shoes and get going! There is really nothing more eco-friendly than walking to a destination. It is nonpolluting, doesn't cost you anything other than your time, and there are numerous health benefits associated with it—a healthier heart, less stress, stronger bones and muscles, and losing and maintaining weight. Walking also gets you outdoors, which is another energy-boosting benefit for your body and your mental health. Here are some opportunities to walk instead of drive:

Get errands done by walking. If it's feasible and you're not carrying home something heavy, try walking to the store. If you're at a strip mall, avoid the temptation to drive closer to your destination after visiting each store—simply walk instead.

Avoid the drive-through. When you're at the bank, fast-food restaurant, or pharmacy, park and walk into the establishment instead of using the drive-through. You'll save fuel and money, and stop emissions dead in their tracks.

Walk your children to school. If the school is less than a mile away, consider walking your children there instead of dropping them off.

Get your cardio the old-fashioned way. Do you drive to the gym, only to get your cardio workout on the treadmill? Fast walk, jog, or run in your neighborhood instead and use your gym for classes or weight lifting.

Bike ☺ ✚

Biking gets you places a lot faster than walking and is a viable method of transportation, especially in urban areas that provide bike lanes, bike garages, bike posts (to chain your bike), and bike rental facilities. And, just like walking, you get all the outdoor benefits and exercise to boost your health. Not only can you bike for leisure and to run errands, you can also make it a serious sport by mountain biking or training for cycling events.

BIKESTATION >> (www.bikestation.org) Urban bike garages available in some U.S. cities where you can park your bike for a small fee while you shop or take care of other errands.

GIANT >> (www.giant-bicycles.com) Extensive line of bikes for all needs; also has a hybrid electric bike that can take you up to 75 miles per charge. If you're looking for a comfortable bike with an around-the-town leisurely feel, check out the Suede Coasting line. The company also has a Web site dedicated to women bike riders, including moms, at www .giantforwomen.com.

MARIN >> (www.marinbikes.com) Company has high-quality bikes for every kind of rider. Its Comfort line of bikes are great for riding around the city or neighborhood; the City line is ideal for commuting; and the ALP series is more for fitness.

SCHWINN >> (www.schwinnbike.com) Carries a full line of bicycles including an electric version that can assist the rider for up to 60 miles; the Collegiate Coasting bike is great for those who have not been on a bike in a while.

Carpool ☺ ✿

Carpooling is not just for work. Connect with other parents who also have to take their kids to school or extracurricular activities. Create a ride-sharing program so that you can save time by not driving to every single event. Think of how much time, gas, and money you'll save!

Consider Public Transportation ✿ $

Public transportation isn't always a flexible or practical option in many areas of the United States because our cities have been built on the principles of urban sprawl. It also can be difficult with smaller children, especially when using a stroller. But if you live in a well-planned urban area that has practical public transportation, consider going carless. You save in gas, do your part for the environment, plus you're able to do other things with your time such as reading, sleeping, or talking with your child. If you live in an urban environment and don't own a car, consider renting, taking a taxi, or enrolling in a car-sharing program for those times when public transportation doesn't cut it.

CARSHARING.NET >> Nonprofit organization that directs you to car-sharing companies and programs in your city.

HERTZ >> (www.hertz.com) While this rental company is known nationwide for their daily rentals, the company recently debuted an hourly rental program in New York City.

ZIPCAR >> (www.zipcar.com) The largest car-sharing program in the nation with service in Atlanta, Boston, Chicago, New York, Philadelphia, Pittsburgh, Portland, San Francisco, Seattle, and Washington, D.C., as well as in London, Toronto, and Vancouver.

make your automobile greener

what you need to know

While a hybrid car can certainly reduce your impact on the environment, you might not be in the financial position to upgrade. Or maybe the current hybrid vehicles don't meet your tastes or needs. Don't despair. There are many things you can do to make your current car greener—some ways are a change in behavior, and other ways involve educating yourself on your fuel options.

benefits

You can save money, reduce emissions, and improve your surrounding environment by changing your driving behaviors and purchasing patterns.

how-to's

Reduce Your Driving ✿ ☺

Did you know a shopping list can make your car greener? Compile a list of items that you will need for the week—groceries, personal care items, dry cleaning—and plan your driving based on the list. This combining of errands will reduce how often you drive. You can also plan a circuit of errands one right after another in the shortest route possible, such as going up to the mall, circling around to the discount department store, and then on over to the nearby grocery store. Additionally, look for chains of stores that are right next to each other to get several errands done at once with the same drive.

Avoid High-Traffic Hours ☺ ✿

You can save yourself a lot of time, money, and headaches—not to mention significantly reduce your car's emissions—by choosing to drive when there is the least amount of traffic. If you have a flexible schedule, avoid traffic and car idling as much as possible.

Improve Your Vehicle's Fuel Efficiency ☺ ✚ $-$$

You want to make the most of the fuel you purchase, which will not only save you money but also reduce your emissions in many cases. Here's how:

Properly inflate your tires: Check your tires at least once a month with a tire pressure gauge to make sure they are inflated to the proper air pressure. The proper air pressure will likely be listed on the inside casing of your driver's door. When your tires are properly inflated, you'll get slightly better gas mileage, be safer on the road, and release less greenhouse gas emissions and air pollutants because of the increase in fuel efficiency. While some tires are more fuel efficient than others, currently no fuel labeling exists. Write to your government officials to request this labeling be made mandatory.

Reduce idling: Turn off your car or park and get out and walk when you might be idling for extended periods. If you idle, you will be burning more gas than it takes to restart your car.

Clean out your trunk: Try to keep your trunk cleared of any unnecessary items. Extra weight makes your car use more fuel.

Drive softly: Avoid fast accelerations and hard braking, which use up extra fuel and expel additional harmful emissions into the air. If you have cruise control, use it to keep your driving smoother on longer, uninterrupted trips, such as on the freeway.

Tune your car: Make sure your car is well tuned, according to your car manufacturer's recommendations. Again, a tuned car will be more fuel efficient and reduce emissions—not to mention the fact that it is safer and more reliable transportation for you and your family.

Change your oil: Get regular service on your vehicle with a periodic oil change, which is usually scheduled based on how many miles you drive. Cleaner oil that lubricates your engine parts will also save on the wear and tear of your vehicle and produce fewer emissions. In most cases, you want to choose synthetic oil instead of petroleum (conventional oil)—unless your car's manufacturer has other guidelines. Synthetic oil doesn't burn off as easily nor cause as much emissions as conventional oil and is often made from a renewable resource like soybeans. Finally, if you or a family member changes your car's oil, the used oil should *not* be disposed of in your trash or poured into the ground. Instead, recycle it according to your municipality's requirements, call 1-800-CLEANUP, or ask your service center if they recycle.

AMSOIL >> (www.amsoil.com) Synthetic automobile oil made from renewable resources.

TRUE FLOW >> (www.trueflow.com) Foam air filters for your car that are washable and reusable over the lifetime of your vehicle; they also provide more air to your engine to boost fuel economy and lower emissions.

Change your air filter: By having a clean quality air filter in your car's system that can trap dust, dirt, and particles which might otherwise get into your car's engine, you'll have better fuel economy and better engine maintenance for your car. Unfortunately, many of the available air filter replacements are paper and polyurethane filters that are not as efficient and are generally thrown into landfills at the end of their short life. They are not reusable and often have reduced performance the more they are used. However, for the environment, your pocketbook, and for performance, whether you change your own filter or have a service do it, look for reusable air filters. These will often be premium filters and will cost you more, but they last *much* longer and are better for the environment—paying back their cost over time.

Open your windows: When you use the air-conditioning in your vehicle, you use more fuel and expel more emissions. Cut down on your AC use by opening your car windows whenever possible.

Slow down on the freeway: Try keeping to the speed limit on the freeway—avoid a lead foot! After sixty-five miles per hour, the fuel efficiency rapidly drops off for most vehicles.

Drive the car that has better gas mileage: If you own two or more vehicles and one gets better gas mileage than the other, choose the better-gas-mileage one to use for the majority of your driving.

Choose Alternative Fuels Whenever Possible ✚ ☺

Your car's fuel options depend on what kind of vehicle you have. Consult your manufacturer guidelines (or inside the fuel-filler door) to know (a) what type of fuel(s) your car will take, such as only gasoline, only diesel, or gasoline and ethanol, and (b) what fuel grade and/or fuel (in the case of a flex-fuel vehicle) is recommended for your engine and fuel efficiency. Flex-fuel vehicles (FFV) can use both traditional gasoline and commonly found gasoline/ethanol blends, as well as higher-ethanol-content fuel blends. Most FFVs can accept higher ethanol blends, like E85. And most diesel vehicles accept a biodiesel blend, like B5 or B20.

When choosing your fuels, keep in mind that some will emit less pollutants into the air than others. There are fuels that are better for our environment as a whole, including how they are produced and manufactured. Currently, there are a growing number of biobased fuels to look into that replace gasoline and diesel fuel, which in many cases reduce emissions and are renewable. They are made from things like corn, sugarcane, or vegetable oil. In order to take advantage of these biofuels, your vehicle has to be either converted or manufactured to use them.

You can do some environmental-benefit comparisons on biofuels based on the kind of crop the fuel comes from and what land is used to grow it on. The best biofuels come from sources that don't compete with food crops, don't destroy native habitats, cause little environmental harm when grown, and have less impact on the environment during the manu-facturing process. Additionally, there are excellent fuel choices available that are neither plant nor petroleum based, such as hydrogen fuel cells and electricity.

The following list, adapted from the Natural Resources Defense Council, shows what the current and emerging fuel choices are on a slid-ing scale of what would be best for your health and the environment.

Best

B100–algal biodiesel: Made from 100 percent algae.

E85–cellulosic ethanol*: 85 percent ethanol mixed with 15 percent gasoline. Made from the cellulose of switchgrass, prairie grasses, cornstalk waste, or other waste materials.

Electricity: This technology is already found in hybrid vehicles.

Hydrogen: An emerging technology, also known as fuel cells.

Close

E85-sugarcane*: 85 percent ethanol mixed with 15 percent gasoline. Comes from the sugarcane plant.

B100–biodiesel: Refined vegetable oil that can be used in nearly any diesel engine. Comes from plants like soybeans, peanuts, and rapeseed (canola). Palm oil is not an eco-friendly source.

SVO: Unrefined straight vegetable oil that can only be used in modified diesel vehicles. Comes from waste oil sources, like leftover restaurant grease.

---

*Can be used in FFVs; E85 has much less emissions, is often better for the environment, and may cost less than other options, but will likely get 20–30 percent fewer miles per gallon than traditional gasoline.

Getting There

E85–corn*: 85 percent ethanol mixed with 15 percent gasoline.

B5 and B20–biodiesel: Refined vegetable oil or algal oil from algae (5 or 20 percent) that is an additive to regular diesel fuel. All diesel vehicles can use this fuel mix.

Natural gas

Beginning to Change

E6 and E10–corn: 6 or 10 percent ethanol mixed with gasoline. You don't have to have a FFV—nearly all nondiesel vehicles can run on this fuel blend.

What to Get Away From

Diesel

Gasoline

sound the ethanol warning bells

There is concern among organizations and activists that the current trend of farming corn for fuel has substantial negative consequences for both the environment and our food stock. Although there are significantly less emissions from corn ethanol fuel blends, corn ethanol is farmed using polluting diesel farm equipment, toxic fertilizers, and large-scale contaminating refinery and distribution processes—only to give us less miles per gallon than gasoline.

On top of this, farming corn for fuel heavily competes for land that was once used to farm corn for human and animal consumption. The result is that our food becomes scarcer and prices go up as food competes for fuel. And according to the Worldwatch Institute, if we wanted to exclusively run our vehicles on E85 fuel, we would have to use 80 percent of U.S. farming land to do so.

Instead of running this risk, there are alternatives to corn ethanol. One is sugarcane, which has 56 percent less greenhouse emissions than gasoline, yields twice as much fuel per acre than corn, and gives you a lot more energy output. But, sugarcane also competes for food and its production and manufacturing process is highly polluting as well.

The best option on the horizon for plant-based fuel is cellulosic ethanol, which is derived from plant fiber and waste. Cellulosic ethanol has a better chance of *not* competing with our food supply and is renewable. It can be made from such things as cornstalk waste, prairie grasses, or other waste materials. When it comes to alternative fuels, write to your state and federal representatives and tell them to give more support to fuels other than corn ethanol, including cellulosic ethanol, algal biodiesel, electric, and hydrogen.

E85 PRICES >> (www.e85prices.com) Shows the difference on a U.S. map of current prices between E85 and gasoline fuels.

NATIONAL ETHANOL VEHICLE COALITION >> (www.e85re fueling.com) Has a U.S. map of where you can buy E85 fuel.

a rush to convert

If you're interested in saving money on gas and significantly decreasing your car's emissions, you might be tempted to convert your car's engine to accept alternative fuels. However, currently no conversion kit or process is certified by the EPA, and most kits are considered do-it-yourself endeavors. These kits contain many unknowns, such as whether or not vehicles that were not manufactured to be flex fuel or run on straight vegetable oil are able to withstand the change in fuel on their internal parts. For example, the hoses and caps might not be able to withstand some of the corrosive elements of a different kind of fuel like E85. Plus, if you convert your vehicle with one of these kits, you may also be voiding any manufacturer or extended warranty.

There are installation specialists associated with some conversion kits, like Greasecar (www.greasecar.com), which offers a straight vegetable oil option for your diesel vehicle. Consult your manufacturer to see if approved conversion kits are available or if a dealership would recommend converting for you, or discuss with a reputable automotive center or installation specialist.

Purchase Eco-Friendly Vehicles ✚ $$$$

When you are ready to purchase a new vehicle, you should consider a greener option. These options include vehicles that:

- Get better fuel mileage.
- Are capable of using alternative fuels (like E85, hydrogen, biodiesel, or electricity); sometimes labeled *hybrid*.
- Are manufactured using greener methods and materials, such as manufacturing facilities that conserve energy and reduce pollution, and materials that come from recycled sources or that last longer.

The best choice is an alternative-fuel vehicle that uses the least amount of fuel of any kind. This could mean a hybrid vehicle with some type of battery inside that is either recharged by simply running the vehicle on the road and/or by plugging in when you get home. Additionally, the new hydrogen-based fuel cell vehicles (FCVs) are an amazing new alternative because they expel very little to no emissions. You can also look for flex-fuel vehicles that allow you to use E85 ethanol. A vehicle with flex fuel and hybrid powering gives you additional refueling options.

Because vehicle technology is evolving so rapidly, you will need to stay abreast of new information and compare and contrast vehicle choices. Before you buy, read reviews, put your best choices and their features side by side, read up on maintenance issues and blog comments by people who already own a vehicle you're interested in, and take a test drive. Remember to look into available tax credits, which can offset such a vehicle's purchase.

EDMUNDS.COM >> (www.edmunds.com) Provides a yearly on-line hybrid buying guide.

FORD >> (www.ford.com) Sells hybrid vehicles under the Ford and Mercury brands.

FUELECONOMY.GOV >> (www.fueleconomy.gov) This EPA Web site is a great tool for comparing vehicles and how they use fuel—efficiently or not. The site also lists what tax incentives are available.

GM >> (www.gm.com) Sells FFV and emerging hybrid options under the Chevrolet, Saturn, GMC, and Pontiac brand names. Many of their vehicles also have what is called active fuel management, which means the car only uses all of its engine capacity when it needs it.

GREEN VEHICLE GUIDE >> (www.epa.gov/greenvehicle) This is an online guide put out by the EPA. You can look up vehicles and make comparisons.

HONDA MOTOR COMPANY >> (www.honda.com) Sells hybrid and fuel-cell technology vehicles. Its FCX Clarity fuel-cell vehicle has *zero toxic emissions* and expels only heat and water.

LEXUS >> (www.lexus.com) Several hybrid vehicle choices including a stylish SUV; Lexus is a division of Toyota.

MAZDA >> (www.mazdausa.com) Sells the Tribute hybrid SUV.

NISSAN >> (www.nissanusa.com) Sells the Altima hybrid.

TOYOTA >> (www.toyota.com) Manufacturer of a variety of a high-quality hybrid vehicles, including an SUV. Toyota is also one of the cleanest vehicle manufacturers, with several of its U.S. plants putting zero waste into landfills.

LIFESTYLE ACTION

be green while on the go

what you need to know

You may have many strategies in place at home to recycle, to buy sustainable and organic products and food, and to reduce your energy and water consumption. But what happens when you're on the go? Sometimes you find yourself in situations where it's difficult to control your greenness, but you should always make an effort! Remember, you don't stop caring about your family outside of your home. And the impact you and your family have on the go is just as important for their health and wellness, as well as for the environment.

benefits

The health of your family, your environment, and communities will be improved by staying green when you are on the go.

how-to's

Recycle Whenever Possible ✚ ∅

When you are on the go, it is inevitable that you will end up with reading material (newspapers, magazines), bottled beverages, and plastic bags or other packaging. In the chance of there not being a recycling bin or container nearby, take a cue from the Boy Scouts and always be prepared . . . for recycling! One easy way is to take it home with you for recycling—you can put the items in a reusable bag in your car and empty it out when you get home. Be on the watch for recycling bins placed in public places.

Avoid Disposable Containers ☺

Plastic water bottles and disposable coffee cups have become ever-present in our society. If you are bringing along food, purchase reusable containers so that you can avoid disposable packaging. Whenever possible, bring a reusable bottle or cup and wash it out when you get home (you may need a bottle brush to get the reusable container completely cleaned). Some coffee shops will even give you a small credit for bringing your own cup. Additionally, it is safer to choose a high-quality aluminum or steel reusable bottle rather than plastic because chemicals from the plastic can leach into your beverage. Ideas are on pages 167–68. If you do choose a plastic water bottle, check that it is labeled PETE (or PET) plastic—also known as plastic #1.

Eat Out Green ✚

There are only a few nationwide chains that are dedicated to green restaurant service. However, many smaller, one-location food establishments throughout the United States are embracing sustainability, organics, and other green restaurant practices; you just have to seek them out, often with an Internet search. When you find them, be a good patron and return—this ensures their success!

These keywords are good signs that the restaurant is taking at least some part of environmental stewardship to heart. If you don't know what exactly the details are, ask some questions about their initiative.

Look for these keywords on the menu or other signage:

> *Biodegradable:* This most likely refers to the takeout packaging, but you want to ask just *how* biodegradable the packaging is. One hundred percent is always best, with no imbedded plastic granules. Biodegradable items can be made from corn, potato, or sugarcane, and straws, napkins, plates, utensils, and cups can be made from these 100 percent biodegradable materials.

> *Chlorine free:* The restaurant is not cleaning or bleaching with chlorine.

> *Conservation:* This is a catchall phrase, just like the words eco-friendly or natural. Find out exactly what they are conserving.

> *Eco-friendly:* This word is a good sign but needs to be backed up with details about *why* the establishment is eco-friendly.

Energy Star appliances: Some or all of the restaurant's appliances are Energy Star–certified, which means that the establishment is using less energy.

Free range, free roaming, cage free: Food labeled with one of these terms is supposed to mean that the animal had been allowed access to the outside. Unfortunately, even with this labeling, there have been widespread abuses of not allowing sufficient access outdoors. Not even "cage free" ensures sufficient access. Look for third-party certifications to verify the company's claims.

Green cleaning: The restaurant is employing green cleaning methods. Hopefully there are additional details in a written policy.

Green power: This may mean the restaurant is powering its establishment with solar or wind power, or that it has converted to using vegetable oil as fuel for indoor appliances. Ask for more info.

Hormone free: This label is important on beef and means the animal was not treated with hormones. (It's already illegal to treat pork or poultry products, including eggs, with hormones.)

Local or family farmed: This probably means less transportation is being used to get the food to your table, and it also may mean the menu changes with the seasons to take advantage of different foods being offered in different growing seasons. Local restaurants also support the organic farming and local farming communities, making a more healthy economic and environmentally supportive cycle of farm to table.

Natural: This term may indicate that further details exist about eco-friendly, sustainable, or organic measures being taken. Under the strictest USDA guidelines, "natural" means that the product contains "no artificial ingredient or added color and is only minimally processed" and an explanation must be provided on the package. For animal products, this label does not offer any indication of how the animal was raised.

Nontoxic: This could mean the use of nontoxic cleaning methods, nontoxic packaging or printing, or nontoxic interior decorating. Ask for details.

Organic: The restaurant is purchasing food that is *certified* USDA 100 percent organic. Ask which foods of the ones they're serving meet this certification.

Recyclable and made from postconsumer recycled waste: All this is good. It may be that your takeout packaging is recyclable and made from recycled materials (such as a certain percentage of postconsumer recycled waste—the higher percentage, the better). Or the establishment may also have recycling programs.

Reduced packaging: Again, it's all about the actual details, but it could mean that your takeout meal has had its packaging reduced so that there is less to throw away, or it could mean that internally the restaurant is choosing suppliers that have reduced their packaging.

Reusable: You are being provided with utensils, cups, napkins, plates, and serving trays that are reusable, such as cloth napkins instead of paper.

Sustainable: The restaurant is purchasing food (seafood or otherwise) from farms or suppliers that engage in growing or fishing practices that enhance the environment and maintain a healthy species.

Water saving: The establishment is somehow saving water, perhaps with its dish washing, bathroom facilities, or cooking methods.

Eat only sustainable seafood: Our oceans are in crisis, due to overfishing, poorly managed fisheries, pollution, and global warming. As a result, each person is responsible for solving these problems by only buying fish that are considered safe, and caught not under siege, in ways that are not damaging to the health of species or habitats. Seafood Watch (www.seafood watch.org) is the best organization to help you find out what is sustainable and safe. More about Seafood Watch and seafood purchasing is found in chapter 6, beginning on page 175.

Look for eco-friendly packaging and serving items: Avoid Styrofoam. Recyclable and biodegradable packaging is the most responsible. There is far too much waste being produced by the restaurant industry, including packaging, napkins, straws, cups, plates, and utensils. Renewable, biodegradable options are your best choices.

CHIPOTLE MEXICAN GRILL >> (www.chipotle.com) Restaurant chain focused on sustainable and healthy food offerings.

PIZZA FUSION >> (www.pizzafusion.com) Has a whole host of environmental initiatives, from the sustainability of the food the establishment serves to how it is delivered; the establishment also tries to source as much of its food as possible from local suppliers.

>> Skip the straw. Since most straws are made from non-biodegradable plastic and aren't necessary for most drinks, help keep plastic out of landfills by refusing or avoiding straws.

LIFESTYLE ACTION
play green

what you need to know

Part of living an eco-friendly lifestyle also means enjoying the earth. When you have the opportunity to appreciate your environment in familiar surroundings, such as at your local park, you and your family are more inclined to care about its maintenance and impact on your community. Being outdoors provides tremendous benefits to your overall mental health and energy for your body, and as long as there are not air quality issues (such as a high ground-level ozone day), being outdoors among the trees and fresh air can have excellent physical benefits as well.

benefits

Local outdoor recreation offers green activities that can save you time and money, encourage environmental stewardship and resource conservation, and give you and your children adequate sunshine, better attention spans, and a more restorative impact on your life.

how-to's

Go Local ✚ ☆ ☺

I always say, "You don't know what you're missing until you move away." For some unexplained reason, a lot of us don't explore what's in our own backyard. But the truth is that it's easier, cheaper, and less stressful on the environment for you to stay local. And playing local is no exception. If you can walk, bike, or use public transportation, then all the better—maybe even making you car-free. Here are some ideas:

> *Local parks:* One fun place to play is your local park. Join your neighbors as they in-line state, play baseball, kick around a soccer ball, or toss a Frisbee around for a few hours. Many parks have recreation departments that offer classes and organized

sports—contact them to see what's available. Your park might also maintain pools, tennis courts, and other facilities where you can have even more fun.

Local schools: Many local schools have free access to their outdoor tracks and fields—yet another place where you and your kids can play and get some exercise.

Local zoo, aquarium, or wildlife center: If you live in or near an urban area, you probably have a zoo, aquarium, or wildlife center close by. They can be wonderful opportunities to relax and learn about nature.

know your air quality

Being outdoors in greenscape boosts your energy and your attention span. Unfortunately, there is only one danger—air quality. Because of all the ground-level ozone and airborne particulates in many of our cities, there can be (especially in the summertime) high pollution levels that make for unhealthy outdoor air. You can check with the Air Now (www .airnow.gov) air quality agency of the U.S. government to check on air quality in your area any time of the year.

Go Outdoors ✚

Today's culture is more focused than ever on staying indoors and it's up to you as a mom to break that cycle for the health and wellness of you and your children. According to the latest research from the University of Maryland, the time children between the ages of nine and twelve spend outdoors has been cut in half between 1997 and 2003—it's gone to a mere 8 percent of their time! This is also combined with the fact that many young children are receiving reduced recess and PE time in their schools (or none at all). And much of this time is replaced with time on the computer, video games, or television. It's not that technology is bad, it's just that there's an imbalance in its overuse. And as a result, you have a whole generation that is growing up disconnected from nature.

So, break this cycle and get outdoors—even if your children initially balk. (Mine do!) Instead of going to the movies, go on a hike together. Require an hour of outdoor playtime every day—even if it means that your child lies down on some grass and watches the clouds go by. Arrange flex time with your work so that you can be home with your kids before the sun sets and you can supervise their outdoor play. During summer vacation, arrange flex time in the mornings so that you can get outdoors with them when the sun comes up—that's the healthiest time to get sunshine. Ask your child's caretaker to make sure outdoor play is part of the day. Encourage outdoor recess and PE at your child's school. Limit screen time from the television, video games, and computer—some operating systems allow you to set timers. Be creative and committed and you'll come up with dozens more ideas.

Here are some quality outdoor activities:

Garden: Gardening provides exercise and relaxation. You can involve the kids, plus it is fun and rewarding to eat the fruits of your labor from your garden.

Cook and eat outdoors: If you have a barbecue or solar oven, cook outdoors. In the summertime, this keeps out unwanted heat from your kitchen.

Exercise outdoors: Recent studies have shown that exercising outdoors amidst a greenscape (as opposed to a strictly urban setting) can be more restorative to your health and boost your brain power. Greenery can clean the air and reduce the temperature around you, both of which are important in the summer months.

Play outdoors: In our wired world, fewer of us are playing outdoors. Why not take a break from TV, video games, and the computer and introduce your kids (and reacquaint yourself) with old-fashioned outdoor play? Ride a bike, take a walk, ride a scooter, jump rope, play hopscotch, draw with chalk on the sidewalk, go horseback riding, water-ski, downhill ski, build a snowman, swim, surf, rake the yard and dive into the leaves, take a hike, rollerblade . . . the outdoor possibilities go on and on and on. If you or your caregiver organizes playdates for your children, meet at a park instead of each other's home.

GREEN HOUR >> (www.greenhour.org) The National Wildlife Federation has a great program called Green Hour that helps you connect your family to nature, and has lots of ideas of how to have fun outdoors with creative and imaginative play. Studies have shown that children and adults who go outdoors for *unstructured* time will likely have less stress, be more physically fit, develop better immune systems, demonstrate fewer attention-deficit problems and be able to more easily focus, and will also create a greater respect and love for the environment.

RAILS-TO-TRAILS CONSERVANCY >> (www.railtrails.org) You can find unused rail corridors that have been transformed into trails through this nonprofit organization.

Visit intriguing outdoor places: Zoos, arboretums, botanical gardens, the beach, or hiking trails.

Camp: You needn't travel far to take advantage of camping opportunities. Chances are there is a state or regional park nearby or you can always camp in your own backyard. Camping provides you with opportunities to play outdoors in surroundings that can be explored. The Leave No Trace (www.lnt.org) program can help you learn how to camp, hike, and enjoy the outdoors with your family in a way that conserves and protects the environment.

technology heads outdoors

If there were ever a super fun way to combine technology with the outdoors, geocaching would be it! Pronounced "geo-cashing," it's a combination of using a mobile GPS (global positioning system) device and going on a treasure hunt to find a "cache"—a hiding place where something is stored. Anyone can hide and maintain a cache. You can find out the coordinates for caches that people across the United States have hidden, from Web sites like Geocaching.com. You input the coordinates into your GPS unit and take off! The coordinates will get you within a few feet of the cache—from there you'll have to hunt around. Once you find the cache, the rules are:

Trade: If you take something from the cache you have to leave something as well. Leave something interesting for the next person, like a foreign coin or stamp, a beautiful landscape picture, a small antique item, inexpensive toys, inexpensive family-friendly CDs or DVDs, money, maps, or books. Also, some caches are themed, like ones with all Star Wars items—so if you don't have a trade item that matches the theme, don't take anything.

Write: You also have to write about your geocaching in the cache's logbook.

Return: You have to return the cache to the exact same spot you found it and in the same or better condition—this also means that if you take something from the cache then what you leave better be of equal or greater value.

Geocaching is just pure fun, especially if you have kids. Since most geocaches are found in the outdoors, it's almost like looking for buried treasure. Geocaching.com also has a Cache in Trash Out program that encourages you to bring along a bag during your geocaching to pick up trash along the way. Have fun!

let's get "more kids in the woods"

The U.S. Forest Service has a More Kids in the Woods program (www.fs .fed.us) that encourages children to experience and connect with the outdoors so that they not only appreciate and enjoy nature but also want to take care of it. Each year there is a related campaign, such as a National Get Outdoors Day in June, to bring attention to this issue.

LIFESTYLE ACTION

vacation with the earth in mind

what you need to know

Travel and tourism is a booming business throughout the world and, as a result, can have an immense impact on the environment and health of the world. It can either promote preservation of our natural and human environment, or degrade it through overdevelopment, overuse of re-sources, destructive waste collection and disposal, and exploitation of people and places that should otherwise be protected.

The good news is that eco-friendly and sustainable tourism initiatives are going mainstream across the globe. As more consumers become more aware of the importance of conservation, they start to question how their travel impacts the world. And the industry is responding—albeit slowly. The most obvious environmentally friendly improvements are recy-cling, but there are other efforts, including water and energy conservation, organic and sustainable food choices, and green building and decorating. For example, some hotels will have water and electricity conservation ini-tiatives for your room and their establishment like the option of not wash-ing your linens every day unless you need it. Many of these travel businesses must work with their government and conservation groups to lessen and limit impact on the natural and human environments—which can be critical in areas that need such things as protection of habitats, beaches, wildlife, and other wild, virgin areas. What all this means for you is learning to travel with the least amount of impact on the environment.

benefits

When you make more eco-friendly vacation choices, your world and health are improved.

how-to's

Choose Green Vacation Places ✚

In the past several years my family has been learning more about nature on our vacations. On one vacation we took a trip to the central California coast to watch elephant seals on the beach—and we were all entranced for hours, even if the seal only moved a few feet. Our guides were volunteer docents and they helped keep the area pristine and undisturbed. The hotel we stayed in supported the local economy and encouraged minimal waste. Vacationing green felt great!

If you're thinking about going on a vacation, look into destinations that offer greener options. And when you're going to spend your money on a trip that is going to cause use of resources and impact the local area (for good or bad), then you owe it to the health and safety of your family—and most certainly the environment and the sustainability of it—to make your best effort to choose more responsible tourism options whenever they exist or your budget allows.

"Sustainable tourism" means that you enjoy all the benefits and beauty of a destination while still minimizing or eliminating the impact of you being there. Unfortunately, there isn't one recognized certification or program to help you choose your destination in a more sustainable way. What is, therefore, most useful is your own research—through simple Internet keyword searches, current travel guides and travel services that focus on green travel or eco-tourism. Whatever the destination, read up on its initiatives and look for transparency about its sustainable tourism efforts. Nearly all destinations will have some Web presence, even if it is through a travel service, so see what they are communicating to you. Here are some additional guidelines of what you should look for:

A written policy about the destination's environmental initiatives, including what it is doing to lessen its impact on or enhance the integrity of the environment, how it's protecting the local wildlife or marine life, and what the vacation destination is doing to improve the lives of the people that live nearby. There should be a list of *details* about what their policy is and its initiatives—nothing should be vague. For example, simply saying "We are dedicated to sustainable tourism" is not enough; again, look for and request substantial details to back that up.

DISNEY >> (http://corporate.disney.go.com) The company's corporate Web site showcases Disney's Environmentality conservation program, which includes a written policy of minimizing and recycling its paper, plant, cardboard, wood, and animal waste. In reducing its greenhouse gas emissions, Disney has introduced cleaner fuel vehicles, promoted ridesharing, and continues to upgrade its buildings for more energy and water conservation.

A verifiable third-party organization affiliation or seal can offer credibility or certification for some or all of the destination's initiatives, including water and energy conservation, and building safety and greenness. For example, in the United States you might see if the destination or accommodations have received the Energy Star certification.

Volunteer opportunities are available for you to get involved in local conservation efforts.

Animals at the destination, such as mules or horses, are taken care of in a humane way and look healthy, and you are able to see how they are taken care of out in the open.

Natural wildlife, surrounding land, and cultures at the destination are not disturbed or altered in order to give you the destination's experience. This should be put in writing.

Employees are not exploited at the destination, and the destination puts its support of its employees and the local economy in writing. Preferably, the destination hires local people for a fair wage.

Independent reviews confirm all that you are reading about the destination. Travel guidebooks, online reviews, and travel services should also be saying the same thing about a destination's overall quality and dedication to sustainability.

vacation in a people- and planet-friendly way

Ron Mader, the founder of Planeta.com, believes in immersion experiences for vacations—travel that helps you understand other people and places and that benefit them and the earth simultaneously.

"As travelers, we have the option of selecting operators and places that show compassion toward the earth," says Mader. He recommends you consider these planet- and people-friendly actions when you vacation:

Pick up the trash: If you are concerned about the environment, show that you care by picking up trash and never throwing anything of yours on the ground.

Learn the language: Learn and use a few words starting with "hello" and "thank you." If you have the time, take a language class.

Be respectful of people's privacy: Some people do not wish to be visited. In rural communities, wait until you are invited to approach homes or groups of people.

Be respectful of restrictions: Some communities may be closed to visitors. Natural attractions might be off-limits for cultural or environmental reasons. When in doubt of whether or not to proceed, ask first.

Be respectful of indigenous people: Traditional land owners should be acknowledged. Aboriginal and indigenous people working in tourism take their role of welcoming visitors very seriously. Recognize their connection to the land and you'll learn to see the world differently.

Buy local crafts: If you are looking for a gift or a souvenir, patronize the arts and demonstrate your support for local culture. Buying from a local artisan can cut out forty steps in the traditional export chain. But *don't* buy items made from endangered animals or pirated archaeological treasures.

leave the golf clubs at home

Not every family vacation has to be a trip somewhere warm to go swimming and golfing. Instead, when planning your next trip, remember that relaxation can include a change of pace, fascinating and useful education, or volunteering. Some of these alternative types of vacations can be done with the kids, while others will probably be a parent's getaway. But they're all worth looking into. Here are some ideas:

Farm vacations: Many of these experiences not only teach you how to tend for plants and animals, but also offer cooking classes to learn how to prepare your harvest. Look into the Pennsylvania Farm Vacation Association (www.pafarmstay.com), the California Agritourism Database (www.calagtour.org), and the Maine Farm Vacation Association (www.mainefarmvacation.com).

Volunteer vacations: Some locations need extra volunteers to do important environmental research or cleanup, reconstruction, or caring for animals. This could be fun and life changing for you and your teenagers. United States-based options include volunteering in restoration programs like Wilderness Volunteers (www.wildernessvolunteers.org) or building projects with Habitat for Humanity (www.habitat.org). Or there are international programs offered at Responsible Travel (www.responsibletravel

.com) including turtle volunteering in the Seychelles, conservation and community projects in the Amazon, and elephant conservation in Thailand.

Little-known getaways: Boost a rural economy that doesn't have the budget of larger destinations or chains. Do your research in magazines like *National Geographic* or *Plenty*, or through eco-travel agencies.

CHARITY GUIDE >> (www.charityguide.org) This nonprofit has a link to a number of environmental volunteer vacation ideas.

CONDÉ NAST TRAVELER >> (www.concierge.com) A travel magazine that often honors and writes about sustainable eco-tourism destinations and services.

EARTHWATCH INSTITUTE >> (www.earthwatch.org) An organization that hooks you and your family up with volunteer opportunities that collect field data for scientific environmental research.

GREEN VACATION HUB >> (www.greenvacationhub.com) Online referral service for green travel and hospitality.

PLANETA.COM >> (www.planeta.com) Online info of all kinds, including articles and resource links, about eco-tourism.

RESPONSIBLE TRAVEL >> (www.responsibletravel.com) Online portal to connect you to more environmentally friendly tourist attractions and travel across the world.

climate change and tourism

At the Second International Conference on Climate Change and Tourism held in Davos, Switzerland, in 2007, it was estimated that tourism contributes about 5 percent of global carbon dioxide emissions. The World Tourism Organization says this includes the emissions of the transportation to get you to your tourist destination, your accommodations, and your activities. By far, airplanes account for more than half of the CO_2 emissions that come from all forms of transport—including vehicles, trains, cruise ships, and any other type of transportation.

Get There Green ✚

Be aware of how you are going to get to your vacation destination. If you have the time, the best choice is by car or train. Air travel is the most polluting—three to seven times more than a car. But if you must fly, take nonstop whenever possible because planes use more fuel to land and take off. You can also reduce travel by staying longer at one destination, as opposed to long distance vacationing several times a year. Try enjoying more short-range or near-home excursions for weekends throughout the year to relax, and then make your real vacation longer. Obviously, all air travel cannot be eliminated, especially if you need to cross oceans. In these cases, look into buying carbon offsets, which counterbalance the CO_2 being released from the airplane (or actually, any energy you use). There are many companies that offer these programs, even some airlines, and the types of green activities that generate these carbon offsets vary. Some include planting trees or the implementation of solar energy.

"in the know" with carbon offsets

Look into carbon offsetting as a way for you to give back to the planet what you take away—in the form of emissions damage to the environment—to ensure your family has a greener and healthier today and future. These emissions may come from your travel, your home, or your business. Carbon offset programs are run by companies or organizations that promise to build windmills, plant trees, or add energy efficiency somewhere.

You should in no way consider carbon offsets to be an environmental pardon when you have other options available that would allow you to reduce your emissions.

Because there is currently little-to-no government oversight, it is up to you to determine which programs are going to be the best investment. Here are some guidelines:

Read the company's Web site carefully: You want to see details and transparency. What is the exact carbon offset project(s)? Are they stating how they'll use your money? Does it seem more like a marketing site? Or is there lots of information from credible sources?

Calculate your emissions correctly: Most carbon offset programs will have a carbon offset calculator on their Web site. Double-check that the calculations add up and are logical.

Look for third-party certification: The best available certification is Gold Standard (www.cdmgoldstandard.org), which requires strict certification and encourages projects that can be audited and measured, such as renewable energy or energy-efficient technologies like wind or solar projects.

Know how your money is used: Look for written transparency from the company stating how much of your money will go directly towards the project. If the carbon offset company is a nonprofit, you can check their rating at Charity Navigator (www.charitynavigator.org). You want to be sure the majority of the money is going to the offset not the administrative payroll.

Make sure it is "additional": Some programs just finance ongoing programs without really increasing carbon offset efforts. Instead, look for the words "add" or "additional" in the carbon offset program information. This means the program is *increasing* carbon offsets.

Avoid forestry projects: These can also be called "sequestration" or "biosequestration" projects, which means the carbon offset program is most likely planting trees. Sequestration projects are controversial in that it is difficult to measure their success. The Gold Standard certification does not support sequestration-only projects. By all means, support forestry projects elsewhere, but look for better programs when it comes to carbon offsets.

CLIMATE FRIENDLY >> (www.climatefriendly.com) Carbon offset program with the Gold Standard third-party verification and a philosophy of reduce, renew, and neutralize.

MY CLIMATE >> (www.my-climate.com) Gold Standard-verified carbon offset program that helps travelers and travel-related companies protect the environment.

NATIVEENERGY >> (www.nativeenergy.com) Multiverified carbon offset program that focuses on building and supporting new, clean, and renewable sources of energy.

TUFTS CLIMATE INITIATIVE >> (www.tufts.edu/tci) Produces reports that analyze and score carbon offset programs.

Look for Eco-Friendly Lodging ✚

Remember to look green when you are looking for a place to stay on your vacation. Many hotels and motels, both small and large, are actively engaging in sustainable and eco-friendly practices. And the best ones will let you know exactly what they are doing—preferably in writing. Interestingly, all the same things you would do at home should be employed in hospitality environments. Here's a list of items you can look for:

Energy efficiency: Conserving of energy with lighting, appliances, electronics, thermostats, and food services; there are Energy Star–certified hotels listed at www.energystar.gov.

Water conservation: Reduction of water usage by encouraging patrons to have their towels and sheets laundered only when needed; aerated faucets and showerheads; low-flow or dual-flow toilets; and other water conservation measures throughout the hotel and in its spa and food services.

ELEMENT HOTELS >> (www.elementhotels.com) This hotel chain uses recycled materials in construction and decor, has Energy Star–rated appliances, has waste-reduction programs, and is pursuing LEED green building certification.

GREEN LODGING >> (www.dep.state.fl.us) A program run by Florida's Department of Environmental Protection that recognizes and rewards environmentally conscientious lodging facilities in the state. There is also a clean boating partnership program and a pollution prevention program.

KIMPTON HOTELS >> (www.kimptonhotels.com) Excellent dedication to eco-friendly hotel practices with its EarthCare program.

MARRIOTT >> (www.marriott.com) International hotel chain has eco-friendly initiatives and goals in energy and water conservation, waste reduction and recycling, and supports community efforts to protect the planet and its habitats. See more at www.marriott.com/environment.

SANDALS AND BEACHES RESORTS >> (www.sandals.com) This resort chain has a written environmental statement, third-party endorsement, and has won awards for its commitment to eco-friendly initiatives.

diy green hotel

You can help to green your hotel by yourself by putting up the Do Not Disturb sign so that your towels and linens won't be washed, or you can make a special request at the front desk. You can also save up your recycling and ask the front desk where to put it, since many hotel rooms don't yet have an in-room recycling can. Also, open your shades or curtains to let in natural light so that you can reduce power use.

Recycling efforts: Recycling bins on the property and in your room; the hotel should be actively recycling internally as well.

Local and organic food: The hotel's food establishment should focus on buying local and organic food.

Green power: Some hotels are now converting to solar power for heating and for electricity. Other hotels may be purchasing from green power sources, like wind power.

Sunshine use: Green accommodations will make use of free sunshine to light your room and other building areas.

Eco-friendly building: The hotel should have been built with the least amount of impact on the surrounding area, and with nontoxic and sustainable building practices whenever possible.

Support of local conservation efforts: If the hotel's location warrants, it should be involved in local conservation efforts of culture, wildlife, land, people, and history; at the very least, every hotel should be involved in improving its local community.

Waste reduction: Composting and wastewater treatment; Styrofoam cups eliminated; electronic information dissemination on your TV screen instead of on paper; and preferably a reduction in overall plastic use, including the elimination of water bottles in the room. Instead, the hotel should offer an in-room water filter and glass cups.

Green cleaning: The hotel should be switching to 100 percent green cleaning from laundering to cleaning your room—no more toxic cleaning and no more chlorine use.

Rent a Hybrid Vehicle ✚

Many car rental agencies are now filling their fleets with hybrid vehicles, so ask for one when you need to rent a car. If you don't own a hybrid, consider this your chance to try one out and do some good for the surrounding air quality and environment.

AVIS >> (www.avis.com) The company is increasing its fleet of hybrid vehicles, along with a large portion of higher-fuel-efficiency vehicles.

ENTERPRISE RENT-A-CAR >> (www.enterprise.com) Has a growing fleet of hybrid vehicles for rent, along with higher-fuel-efficiency vehicles.

HERTZ >> (www.hertz.com) Has higher-fuel-efficiency and hybrid rental vehicles available, including Toyota Priuses.

Try a Homebased Vacation ⚙ ☺

The farther your vacation destination, the more pollution you will cause. Consider taking a homebased vacation, also called a "Staycation." This requires a bit of discipline to disconnect from your errands and work, but it can be quite relaxing. After all, you don't have to deal with the hassles of traveling, and you get to sleep in your own bed. Here are some tips:

Treat it just like a regular vacation: Tell everyone that you'll be gone, and disconnect from e-mails, work, phones, and errands.

Plan out what you want to do: Treat it just like a regular vacation. Whether you want to just bum around the house or explore local tourist attractions, know ahead of time what you want to be doing so that you can make it easier to disconnect.

Make it fun and interesting: Time to be a tourist in your own hometown! Check out the local zoo, botanical garden, arboretum, amusement park, aquarium, beach, state park, art show, car show, city park, hiking trails, horseback riding stables, special events and concerts, movies—whatever you like to do. Your local newspaper should have a wealth of information about special events as well. Just think about disconnecting and letting go.

the green-collar workforce: an earth-friendly influence in the office

These days, most environmentalists will tell you that we've got to start farther "upstream" to take care of our planet, our safety, and our health. What they are referring to is the notion that manufacturers and businesses need to take more responsibility for improving use of resources, stopping pollution, making products that have zero waste, and eliminating product toxicity as opposed to everyone else trying to clean up the mess after the fact. If you're a working mother, you can be at the beating heart of this change at the office. If you have decision-making power, go for the gusto when it comes to making green choices. And when it comes to everyday personal decisions, such as those about your commute, there are always more eco-friendly and cost-effective choices.

LIFESTYLE ACTION
be a green boss

what you need to know
If you own your own business or are in a position to make policy and/or purchasing decisions at work, you have a platform from which you can help your company become more green. When businesses become more environmentally friendly, it can have a tremendously positive effect on the earth—especially when it comes to product manufacturing. So much waste, pollution, and negative environmental impact come from a product or service's source—the supplier or the manufacturer.

It's time to shift our focus from managing waste, cleaning up toxic messes, and dealing with health concerns to stopping it all at the source. If you manufacture and supply in a sustainable manner, you ensure that your business has a more viable future. And know that your business's environmental policies don't have to be dry; you can be green and have fun at the same time. For example, have an Energy Fair to help your employees learn more on a broadscale, offer green contests, e-mail fun reminders, and give gift certificates for reaching goals.

benefits

Your and your family's health can be improved and our natural resources can be conserved if you encourage your business to become champions of the environment in everything they do and create. You are also planning for your business' future when you ensure that your practices, products, and services are sustainable.

> **GREENBUSINESS.NET >>** (www.greenbusiness.net) This is a helpful online forum for networking and finding out how other businesses are going green.

eco-mizing your business works

Patricia Calkins, vice president of environment, health, and safety at Xerox Corporation (www.xerox.com), says, "Many organizations today still struggle to justify a meaningful investment in green initiatives, because they perceive the efforts will generate added costs, not concrete business benefits." But the reality is that "case studies from virtually every industry show that it's possible for businesses today to develop green initiatives that will make a quantifiable contribution to both the environment and the bottom line."

For example, when you upgrade to more energy-efficient office equipment, you do have a cost for the upgrade, but the investment will not only save you money in the long run but also have a positive environ-mental impact. Additionally, it's important to remember that a com-pany's greening efforts may also bring along added benefits of improved employee morale, customer loyalty, and a solid positive brand image—all this affects a business in a positive way.

how-to's

Buy and Supply Responsibly ✚

One of the best ways your company can go green is by buying and sup-plying more responsibly. Start with office products and green cleaning. I've presented many ideas and resources in the earlier chapters of this book, as well as the school section of chapter 9.

From there, look at what your business produces and how you can choose greener suppliers and supplies—choose nontoxic, low-energy use, nonpolluting, recycled, sustainable, and organic, to name a few. Look into sourcing more green raw materials for manufacturing, such as those that come from recycled sources. Hewlett Packard (www.hp.com) is a good example; the company has been making new inkjet cartridges out of 70–100 percent recycled plastic. Throughout chapter 6 there are additional guidelines on green purchasing that are invaluable to under-standing your best options in the marketplace.

ARAMARK >> (www.aramark.com) Food services for businesses and schools. Offers environmental stewardship guidelines, runs a reusable lunch bag program, and is a Seafood Watch (www.sea foodwatch.org) partner.

BON APPÉTIT MANAGEMENT COMPANY >> (www.bamco .com) A food service company with on-site corporate and educa-tional institution services as well as off-site catering. The company is dedicated to sustainable, responsible, and healthy food options.

(continued)

FORESTETHICS >> (www.forestethics.org) A nonprofit action organization that protects endangered forests and has a number of tools and resources online to help you implement a forest-friendly purchasing policy.

RESPONSIBLE PURCHASING NETWORK >> (www.responsible purchasing.org) Has many resources for companies to learn more about and link into for more responsible and environmentally friendly purchasing, procurement, supplier sourcing, and products.

OFFICE OF THE FEDERAL ENVIRONMENTAL EXECUTIVE >> (www.ofee.gov) This White House task force on waste prevention and recycling has an informative green purchasing section on its Web site and also includes a link to a paper calculator (www.papercalculator .org), which can help you compare individual types of paper or paper categories. By comparing your paper choices, you can learn which decisions can impact the environment more positively and manage resources more wisely. Results compare:

Amount of virgin wood required to meet your needs.

Total energy expended to produce the paper.

Greenhouse gases released when paper is manufactured using fossil fuels and when it decomposes in landfills, giving off methane.

Wastewater, which includes the measurement of fresh water needed to manufacture the paper as well as wastewater impact.

Solid waste, which includes the sludge and other wastes produced through manufacturing.

Deliver Green ✚

If your business is one of millions that delivers products or mail to customers, look for greener ways to do it. For example, avoid Styrofoam and reduce packaging. Other ideas include:

Avoid petroleum plastic: Whenever possible, avoid petroleum plastic altogether. But, if you must use it, look for new-technology, agriculture-based plastics that will biodegrade fully without any petroleum plastic granules leftover.

Look for nontoxic packaging: Use packaging that contains no PVC or other toxic chemicals.

Use recycled materials: Purchase recycled paper, printer ink, toilet paper, envelopes, mailer bags, and paper towels.

Choose 100 percent biodegradable: Look for packing or packaging that will fully biodegrade with no petroleum plastic granules leftover. You can call or e-mail a company to find this information out for sure, if it is not listed on the company's Web site or marketing materials. The makers of some new corn-based plastics promote that they come from renewable resources but do *not* offer biodegradability or offer only limited and labor/energy-intensive biodegradability with no chance of biodegrading in the ocean or on the side of the road. Also, the companies making these products make no effort to consider organic farming. *Avoid these products and look for better options.*

Select reusable options: Packaging for shipping can be reusable, such as envelopes that can be turned inside out and used again.

Offer your customers ground shipping options: Air shipping creates much more pollution than ground shipping.

ever consider compostable packaging?

Packaging that gives back to the earth is a new concept that's taking hold. Jardine Foods (www.jardinefoods.com), operating out of Austin, Texas, uses 100 percent biodegradable packing peanuts and bubble wrap packaging. Since the peanuts are made out of cornstarch and are 100 percent biodegradable, you can throw them into the compost pile. And although the bubble wrap is made from polyethylene, it has an eco-friendly additive that, in one year's time, breaks down the wrap into pieces that are small enough for microorganisms to eat. The wrap is then turned into water when it is composted by the microorganisms; they essentially secrete water after having eaten what was formerly the wrap. Polyethylene without this additive would virtually never break down. Finally, the boxes for their products and packing materials are completely recyclable and the boxes contain a note (printed on 100 percent recycled paper) that explains what to do with the bubble wrap and packing peanuts.

canon packages green

Canon (www.usa.canon.com), the manufacturer of printers and printer cartridges, has developed a Generation Green initiative to reduce energy and resource use and be environmentally friendly with its products and manufacturing. One of the results of the program is that select ink packs are being packaged with biodegradable limestone packaging, which reduces the need for paper and other raw materials. The company says that using biodegradable packaging causes "a 45 percent reduction in natural energy, 65 percent reduction in petroleum-based plastics, and 50 percent reduction in emissions that impact global warming."

BIODEGRADABLE PRODUCTS INSTITUTE >> (www.bpiworld .org) Has a certification program to identify plastic products that will biodegrade and compost. There is an approved product list online.

EARTHSHELL >> (www.earthshellnow.com) 100 percent biodegradable plates and bowls made from corn, potatoes, and limestone that can be used for food delivery.

ECO-PRODUCTS >> (www.ecoproducts.com) Eco-friendly, sustainable, and nontoxic food service supplies.

FEDEX >> (www.fedex.com) Has a ground shipping option, as well as reusable envelopes.

PELICAN >> (www.pelican.com) The company sells virtually indestructible, reusable plastic cases that can be used to pack and ship back and forth nearly indefinitely, cutting down on Styrofoam and cardboard use.

STALK MARKET >> (www.stalkmarket.com) Biodegradable and 100 percent compostable disposable paperware and flatware.

STARCH TECH >> (www.starchtech.com) 100 percent biodegradable peanut packing material made from corn and potatoes with no petroleum.

STOROPACK >> (www.storopackinc.com) Variety of environmentally friendly packing materials available with no petroleum plastics in the materials.

TREECYCLE >> (www.treecycle.com) Sells recycled paper, eco-friendly office and cleaning products, and biodegradable food service products.

UPS >> (www.sustainability.ups.com) Besides providing a ground-shipping service, the shipping company is serious about addressing environmental issues—including operating the greenest vehicle

(continued)

fleet in the shipping industry, using less trucks (equaling less pollution) to deliver, and reusable next day air envelopes which are
bleach free and made from 100 percent recycled fiber.

Print Responsibly ☺ ✿ ✚

Most businesses do a lot of printing—either in-house by printing off
pages from the computer or through their marketing campaigns. This
can be incredibly wasteful, not to mention toxic, if you consider chemicals that may have gone into the ink and the likely use of virgin resources (virgin paper). Look for ways to cut down on using paper. The
best choice is to avoid printing altogether. One way to do this is by dis-
seminating information about your company by e-mail or on the Internet.

For example, you can make electronic brochures available via your
company's Web site instead of on paper. But if you have to print on paper, use paper with the highest percentage of recycled and postconsumer waste available and use soy ink. Although paper is biodegradable
and can come from renewable resources, according to the Bureau of International Recycling, recycled paper manufacturing creates over 70
percent less air pollution and about 35 percent less water pollution
when compared to virgin paper manufacturing (making paper from
wood). The environmental and health benefits are significant enough for
you to choose recycled over virgin paper. But, if any percentage of the
paper you are printing on is virgin paper (directly from a tree and not recycled), then be sure the virgin paper is certified by the Forest Stewardship Council (FSC) as being taken from a responsibly managed forest.
Also, choose paper that was processed without chlorine, to reduce toxicity in wastewater. Some acronyms to look for:

PCF (Processed Chlorine Free) means that the product was not
processed with chlorine or chlorine compounds—this acronym is
largely used on paper products with recycled content.

ECF (Elemental Chlorine Free) means that although the paper was bleached, it was done using alternative chlorine compounds, which reduce harmful by-products.

TCF (Totally Chlorine Free) means that your product was processed with no chlorine. TCF is largely used on paper products from virgin fiber.

the difference between recyclable, recycled, and postconsumer waste

With all the earth-friendly terms flying around out there, it can sometimes be confusing. And even though you see a universal recycle symbol on the package, you can read more on the label for clarity. When it comes to purchasing products, here are three terms that you should be clear about:

Recyclable: This means the product can be recycled.

Recycled: This means the product came from a percentage of recycled, nonvirgin materials. The best labeling says more than "recycled" and instead states the percentage that is recycled, like, "made from 100 percent recycled materials." Recycled materials can be preconsumer waste, postconsumer waste, or a mix of both.

Preconsumer waste: This means that the product came from a percentage of waste that has not yet gone through the consumer waste stream. For example, paper can be made using paper scraps and trimmings from a paper factory.

Postconsumer waste (sometimes labeled PCW, or PCC for postconsumer content): This means that the product came from a percentage of waste that has already been used by consumers and is now being brought back to the manufacturing process to be used again. Seek products with the highest amount of PCW possible, because that means less new materials are being used to create the product.

Here's an example—if you see a product that says "50 percent recycled, 20 percent PCW," then this means (and you have to do a little math):

- Since only 50 percent was recycled, the other 50 percent is virgin (paper made directly from trees, not recycled paper).
- The 50 percent recycled is composed of 20 percent postconsumer waste (PCW).
- By deduction, then, the other 30 percent must be preconsumer waste.

Here's another example—"100 percent recycled, 40 percent PCW." This means:

- All of the product comes from recycled materials.
- Of that 100 percent, 40 percent is postconsumer waste.
- The other 60 percent is preconsumer waste.

THE FOREST STEWARDSHIP COUNCIL >> (www.fscus.org) This important organization sets standards and criteria for responsible forestry across the globe, as well as certifies both forests and forest products (like wood or paper products). A product bearing the FSC label has been sourced from a well-managed forest that follows FSC's standards.

the many benefits of soy ink

Regular ink is made from petroleum. Soy ink, however, is made from soybeans. The advantages of soy ink over petroleum ink are many:

- Low in VOCs, which means that significantly fewer harmful gases and emissions occur.
- Minimal toxic waste.
- Brighter colors.
- Less ink is required to print the same number of pages.
- Can be used by a laser printer.
- A renewable resource.
- Easier and nonhazardous to remove when paper gets recycled.

Conserve Energy ☺ ✚

Energy conservation at work happens by setting policies at your business that not only change how people do things and how products and services are made and delivered, but also what is purchased. Here are some of the ways your business can conserve energy:

Obtain a professional energy audit on your business: This will give you direction and a checklist, of sorts, on how your business can save energy. The consultant who performs the audit may also be able to help you determine how much money you would be saving if you upgraded to more energy-efficient options; this can be helpful for figuring out a budget.

Become Energy Star compliant: Set a policy that your company will phase out any appliances and related supplies that are not Energy Star compliant. This includes computers, printers, lighting, heating, and cooling. Make sure any phased-out supplies and appliances are either donated to a good cause (school or nonprofit) or sent to the proper recycling facility. See more about Energy Star and energy conservation in chapter 3.

Program all electronics to standby: Many Energy Star computers, printers, and other electronics have a standby or sleep setting that powers down to minimum energy use after a number of minutes of nonuse. Set a policy that all such electronics be programmed with standby mode.

Buy green power: Purchase greener power options and set goals for increasing the percentage of green power purchased over time. Wind power is becoming a popular green power. Read more about green power in chapter 3.

Turn off the lights: Many businesses and their buildings leave lights on in the evening or in rooms that are not in use. Your business can save money immediately by turning off the lights at night and installing motion sensors in all rooms so the lights turn off automatically when not in use.

EARTH HOUR >> (www.earthhour.org) A campaign by the World Wildlife Fund (www.wwf.org) that encourages residents and businesses to turn off their lights when not in use. Every year there is a promotional earth hour when everyone across the globe is encouraged to flip their switches to "off" to send a message about climate awareness.

Avoid business trips whenever possible: With video and telephone conferencing, you can not only save your business a lot of money, but also reduce travel's toll on the environment and your employees' health by staying at the office for meetings instead of flying or driving.

Change to more energy-efficient lights: Although you need as much natural light and daylight lighting as possible during your workday so your energy can be kept up and you can see your work more easily, your business can make a policy of phasing in more energy-efficient lighting. Install sunlights (a highly energy-efficient option) or fluorescent daylight lighting, which will also save money. Energy Star lighting fixtures are also great investments for saving energy.

THE VISTAWALL GROUP >> (www.vistawall.com) Has beautiful skylights that will not only save you money on energy by lighting your business with the sun, but will also add beauty to your building.

>> Research shows that brighter light, like that of daylight lighting or sunlight through skylights, can increase employee performance by up to 20 percent.

Take notice of your landscape: Your company's landscape can be helping or hindering the heating and cooling energy costs. See how the trees and bushes around your business' property may assist you in conserving power.

>> Institute a carbon offset program to make up for the emissions your company produces. This is good environmental policy and contributes to the sustainability of your business. See chapter 7, page 212 for information on buying certified carbon offsets.

windblown and loving it

One company that has taken green power to heart is Aveda (www .aveda.com), which has the distinction of being the first beauty company to be manufacturing its products with 100 percent wind power. Aveda purchases the wind-produced power from its utility company Xcel Energy (www.xcelenergy.com), currently available in eight U.S. states.

Conserve Water ☺

Just as your company should conserve energy, it should also conserve water—largely by upgrading your building's systems and fixtures that use water. Here are some ideas:

Upgrade to water-efficient fixtures and toilets: Save your company money by phasing in upgrades to your faucets and toilets. Have a plumber install aerators on your faucets and also consider investing in low-flow and dual-flush toilets, as well as faucet replacements. There are some faucets that have motion sensors, which can be an excellent choice in a public place. Chapter 2 has lots more info on water-efficient fixtures and toilets.

Improve your property's landscaping water use: Landscaping is another area in which your company can save water. Phase in more native plants that use less water, as well as upgrade your watering system with drip irrigation or a weather-tracking feature. See chapter 5 for more ideas.

Upgrade to water-efficient appliances: If your business uses water for dish washing or other purposes, consult with your appliance or product distributor about upgrading to more water-efficient systems. If upgrading isn't an option, look at your processes to determine how you could save water using your same system.

Encourage Recycling ✚ ☺

No matter how green your business is, chances are you will still have a great deal to recycle. Depending on the size of your company, put a committee together which can help:

- Audit all the items that are currently being thrown away and recycled.
- Review the audit and create guidelines for increasing the recycle rate; look for ways items can be reused.

- Identify what your current waste company or city sanitation department can or cannot do with waste and your recycling initiatives.
- Research ways your company can receive money back for recycling, such as through reverse vending machines or through an agreement with an outside recycler.
- Look into ways your company could donate items and collect a tax deduction (instead of recycling or throwing away)—for example, computer equipment and unused letterhead and paper could be donated to schools. Additionally, you can provide recycling of your products at the end of their lifespan to your customers—for example, if you're in the carpet business you can accept your customers' old carpets and recycle them into another type of sellable product.
- Provide annual reports of green goals met as a true statement of environmental responsibility.

Additionally, the EPA has a WasteWise program (www.epa.gov/wastewise) that can assist your organization in finding more ways to prevent waste, recycle, and purchase recycled waste.

Clean Green ✚ ☺
The health and happiness of your employees is vitally important to not only your bottom line but also for their overall well-being. As a result, look into instituting a policy that your business will only clean green. Chapter 4 and the school section of chapter 9 have excellent material and resources for you to develop your policy.

Give Back to the Community ✚ ☺
Businesses have the ability to finance many community endeavors with eco themes. The benefits to your business are huge:

- Increased public and shareholder support for your business.
- Improved name recognition.

- Opportunity to connect "doing the right thing" with your company or product's name, such as in a sponsored event or initiative.
- Security of your community's health and sustainability, including protecting your employees' way of life and health—this has huge bottom-line residual effects.
- Tax deductions for giving to nonprofits—choose nonprofits that benefit the community's health, safety, and environment.

You can do good in small or large projects—whether through schools, city programs, or nonprofit organizations.

ikea's plant-a-tree program

In line with IKEA's (www.ikea.com) environmental commitment is its partnership with the American Forests organization (www.american-forests.org) to offset the CO_2 emissions produced by IKEA employees and visitors driving to its stores each year. They are doing this by planting about 33,100 trees each year through American Forests' Global Re-Leaf program in what is called IKEA's Plant-a-Tree initiative. Trees "inhale" carbon dioxide, absorbing the harmful carbon, and then "exhale" clean oxygen back into the air. This is just one of the many ways IKEA is giving back to the community at large.

EARTH SHARE >> (www.earthshare.org) An organization that can help your business set up programs to support environmental initiatives.

LIFESTYLE ACTION

green your commute

what you need to know

Americans make up only about 5 percent of the world's population, yet own nearly a third of all automobiles, guzzling more than 400 million gallons of gasoline per day. Commuting to work accounts for a big chunk of that fuel usage, and nearly 80 percent of us who drive to work are alone in our vehicles. Nearly all of us would love to hop across the street to get to the office, so long as our residential living was uncompromised. But that isn't the case for most people. The reality is that for your health and environment, you need to find ways to change the way you travel to work in order to decrease the amount of pollution expelled in the process.

benefits

You can improve air quality, reduce waste, conserve energy, and even save some money by greening your commute.

how-to's

Live Closer to Work ✚ ✿ ☺

When we lived in the Phoenix, Arizona, area, we saw urban sprawl take hold in a very big way. There was a building boom, and many people jumped at the chance to own a much larger home for less at the expense of living farther away from work. This created more traffic problems and, in turn, a need for more freeways. The brown haze (hazardous ground-level ozone) thickened each morning and evening throughout the metro area as more and more people drove more often and farther to get to work. The major problems with all this sprawl, which is a common occurrence in many cities across the United States, include:

- More pollution in your air and environment.
- More driving expense and fuel use, which isn't good for the environment or your pocketbook.

- More time away from your family, which also equals more stress.

Yes, you need safety and good schools and good quality of life, but if it is at all possible to live closer to work, then do it.

Choose Alternative Transportation ✚ ✿ ☺ $–$$

There are over a hundred cars parked every morning at the local commuter train stop in my city. While they could drive, these commuters are saving themselves at least an hour in traffic by using the train. They're also saving money, improving air quality, and lowering their stress. Follow their lead and try these alternative transportation options to get to work:

Walk: If your work is less than a mile away from home, put on a comfortable pair of shoes and walk. Imagine the exercise you'll get, plus the money you'll save on gas!

Bike to work: Depending on your type of work and the weather, this could be an option; however, if you're a stiletto gal in a suit, this is probably not the best choice.

Carpool: This can definitely save you money, and on the days you're not assigned to drive you can read or work on your laptop. Some workplaces encourage carpooling and will help you find other employees who live in your area and are willing to carpool.

Use public transportation: If there is a train, bus, or subway with a schedule and route that is convenient for you, look into it. Public transportation can give you opportunity to read, work, or do other tasks on your way to your job; plus you'll save money and possibly time spent in traffic.

Telecommute ✚ ✿ ☺

If your job allows you to work part- or full-time from your home, you might want to consider telecommuting. With the right discipline and at-home work environment and equipment, you can prove quite efficient with the commute being from your bed to the computer.

Ask for Flextime ✚ ✿ ☺

Some jobs allow for flextime, which means you have a variable work schedule. For example, one day you might come in at 11 A.M. and leave at 7 P.M. and the next you might work from 8 A.M. to 6 P.M. You are allowed to manage your work time yourself, as long as your work gets done. This can be very healthy for you and for the planet, because you are able to commute during nonpeak traffic hours (which means less idling on the road) and you are able to reduce your stress because less commuting time means more ability to get things in your life done (like doctor visits, gardening, or exercising in the morning). In some jobs you can ask for a combination of flextime and telecommuting as long as your productivity and performance are not compromised.

LIFESTYLE ACTION

green your desk

what you need to know

Even if you aren't the boss, you can still take steps to go green at work. These are personal choices that you can make regardless of office policies or tedious bureaucracies. And with you spending a third or more of your day at the office, it is really important to treat it like a home away from home and go green every day.

benefits

You can improve your air quality, reduce waste, and conserve energy by making personal green choices at work. Many of these choices also keep more money in your bank account and improve the quality of your life.

how-to's
Bring Your Own Lunch ☺

If you bring your own lunch (remember—in reusable containers) on most days of the week, you will save a bundle. It's easy to spend ten dollars or more on a lunch each day, and that's a cheap lunch that may or may not include a drink—plus there's all the waste that's produced by a purchased lunch. Conversely, a lunch brought from home can cost you only half that much or less—especially if you've brought leftovers.

Eat Out Green ✚

There's often no escape from business lunches as they are a part of work politics and social conventions. So look in chapter 7, beginning on page 197, for ideas on how to eat out greener.

Drink from Reusable Cups ☺

Stop the disposables in their tracks by drinking from a reusable cup whenever possible—for water and coffee. If you need some mobility, use an aluminum container as it is not only durable but also completely recyclable at the end of its life.

Choose Your Coffee Carefully ✚ ☺ $

We're a nation addicted to caffeine and as coffee chains have popped up in every city and town in recent years, the addiction is growing. Coffee once grew under tree canopies (shade grown) but as the market for coffee grew, farmers cleared the trees and planted sun-grown varieties. As a result, countless rain forests and bird habitats have been destroyed, creating devastating consequences for the environment. Additionally, many coffee laborers do not receive fair wages. And last but not least is the problem of waste in the form of disposable coffee cups. Well-known coffee chains are not doing enough to reverse harmful effects on the environment related to coffee. Instead, here's what you can do to force change:

Only buy coffee that is triple certified: shade grown, certified USDA organic, and fair trade certified. If your coffeehouse isn't providing you with this option, give the store manager a verbal or written request; if you have limited options, at least go with shade grown because it has multiple environmental benefits (less fertilizer use, restores habitats, helps stem global warming because of the trees, decreases soil erosion) as well as more flavor due to a longer growing cycle.

Use a reusable cup: Ask your coffeehouse if it will fill your reusable cup instead of using a disposable cup.

Bring your own coffee from home: Prepare your eco-friendly coffee at home and bring it to work in your reusable cup.

BIRD-FRIENDLY SEAL >> (www.si.edu/smbc) Shade-grown certification by the Smithsonian Migratory Bird Center to help protect migratory birds and their habitats.

THE CENTER FOR A NEW AMERICAN DREAM >> (www.newdream.org) Resource for and supporter of fair-trade, shade-grown, organic coffee.

GROUNDS FOR CHANGE >> (www.groundsforchange.com) Sells coffee that is fair-trade certified, shade grown, and certified organic.

TRADER JOE'S >> (www.traderjoes.com) Sells fair-trade coffees, with shade-grown certified-organic varieties.

TRANSFAIR USA >> (www.transfairusa.org) Independent, third-party certifier of fair trade products in the United States.

(continued)

WHOLE FOODS >> (www.wholefoodsmarket.com) Sells a variety of more eco-friendly coffees.

Reduce Your Paper Use ☺

It's crazy how much paper businesses can go through. They often print like there's no tomorrow. But, no matter what your employment position, there are things you can do to reduce paper use:

Choose to go paperless whenever possible: Instead of printing things out, send an e-mail with electronic attachments. If your company allows, end your e-mail with the signature line "Please consider the environment before printing this e-mail."

Make double-sided copies: Copy on both sides of the paper instead of just one to immediately reduce your paper use by 50 percent; if possible, set the printer to print double sided.

Proofread on the screen: If you feel your accuracy isn't hampered, proofread your documents on the computer instead of printing them out.

Use scrap paper: Keep a scrap paper file and use it for anything that doesn't require the public's eye, such as internal business meetings or notepaper.

Turn Off or Standby ☺

Turning the switch to "off" or "standby" for electronics is the same at work as at home. Look for opportunities to turn off the power of your computer or lights. You can also set your computer to go into standby after ten minutes of not using it.

>> American businesses could save over $1.7 billion per year by having their employees shut off their computers at the end of the day.

Do Your Own Recycling Drive ☺

If your company isn't doing all the recycling it can and you have permission from your boss, bring recyclable items from work to a recycling facility or another recycling program yourself.

CHAPTER NINE

your green community: care about important issues ... and do something about them

You know that growing your family green starts at home and that your green actions should stem outward—to your shopping, to your travels and recreation, and to your work. But what about the community at large? Your community, including schools, is the foundation of your life and our future, so a lot is at stake. Because your children likely spend more than half of their waking hours at school, you owe it to their health and to the environment to treat your child's school like a second home. Luckily, what you have learned about your home and garden earlier in this book are templates for school.

Additionally, if you don't take care of the other parts of your community, you will sacrifice the health and safety of you and your family and will experience a reduced quality of life. The only way to ensure that your community will be taken care of in a sustainable and healthy way is to make people care. Our governments are run by people. Our laws are established by people. And it is people who make or break our environment. In all of this, one person can truly make a difference—this is one point that you should never forget.

LIFESTYLE ACTION
be a force of change in schools

what you need to know

When I sense that something needs fixing at my child's school, I usually just pick up the phone and ask to speak to the principal or counselor. Although I am diplomatic and positive, I'm also action minded. Sometimes there is a protocol, such as working through a parent organization or going to a board meeting. Other times you simply need to take the initiative.

Most schools are not yet going to come right out and tell you what efforts they are taking to become green. So, you're going to have to ask questions—in the nicest way possible, of course. And then once you know what they are or are not doing, you can determine how you would like to go about working on some improvements. No matter what method you use (and I name many ways in this chapter) to help your child's school be more environmentally friendly, safe, and healthy, you'll need to understand that it will take some of your time. Schools are short on staff and money, so you may need to research, volunteer, and hold fundraisers. Because of this time commitment and because working with others can yield better and faster results, I recommend pairing up with like-minded moms whenever possible.

benefits

Your child's health, safety, and well-being can be significantly improved if his/her school makes more eco-friendly decisions about their purchases and practices. Moreover, since schools are catalysts for change in the community, your actions can help the environment on a larger scale.

eco-fundraising

Many of today's school fundraisers are about buying more junk or junk food. Instead, why not green your school's fundraiser? Here are some ideas:

Water bottle collection: If your state pays for returning water bottles, do a water bottle collection and reap the financial benefits.

Selling unclaimed lost-and-found items in an annual fundraiser, including any leftover items found in school lockers at the end of the school year.

CHICOBAG FUNDRAISER >> (www.chicobag.com) Sell these reusable bags as a fundraiser; you can even have the bag imprinted with a school logo.

FUNDING FACTORY (www.fundingfactory.com) A printer cartridge and cell phone recycling program to be used as a fundraiser.

GREENRAISING (www.greenraising.com) Provides products for school fundraising that helps families consume less, preserve natural resources, and help others.

REUSABLE PLANET (www.reusableplanetonline.com) Schools can raise money by collecting empty printer cartridges and also by providing refilled printing supplies for purchase.

WAL-MART KIDS RECYCLING CHALLENGE: (www.kids recyclingchallenge.com) A program that teaches elementary school students about the importance of recycling while earning money for their schools.

how-to's

Create a Green School Action Blueprint ✚ ✿ ☺

One of the best ways to be a force for change in your child's school is to get organized. Determine what it is that you wish to focus on, what questions you want to ask, and what research needs to be done. This will save you time and money in your volunteer work and will help you get the results you seek.

The following is a Green School Action Blueprint to help you brainstorm and start thinking about both the issues your child's school may be facing and ideas for improvement. What you have learned in the previous sections about going green in your home, your garden, and in the marketplace is applicable in your child's school; you just have to apply those lessons on a larger scale and within a bureaucratic system. Virtually no school is ideal when it comes to environmental and health issues. But you can influence and jump-start change. Here's how you might tackle this blueprint so you don't feel overwhelmed:

Read through the issues presented in the blueprint list.

If you want to confront an issue on your own, determine which one most interests you. Focus on researching and volunteering to make solutions happen over time. There are suggestions in the how-to portion of this section later in this chapter. Make sure you have enough time to make your effort a success.

If you want to work with other like-minded parents on one or more issues, look at the suggestions in the how-to portion of this section to see how you might coordinate your ideas and efforts with others so that each person can do his and her part. Sometimes working together can make change happen more quickly and lend additional strength of voice and interest. Working with others also allows for the good use of multiple talents and skills and (if needed) can contribute contacts for fundraising and donations.

As you traverse this list and begin to think of your own ideas, there are some other important things to remember:

Schools are budget conscious. Any *cost savings* that you can offer will get change happening faster.

Schools are time conscious. Any *time* you can volunteer to help make something happen will make your idea more palatable.

Schools are liability conscious. So if money savings aren't motivation enough, move to Plan B; talk about the costs, particularly in terms of health dangers, that the system will incur if change doesn't happen. But be careful with this approach, because you don't want to create enemies, especially if there isn't any budget in place for your project. Position yourself as someone who wants to help the school find solutions. If they buy into the importance of an idea, then even if the school or school district doesn't have money, they will work with you to find other ways to fund an initiative—such as through fundraising, grants, or corporate sponsors.

>> This blueprint is written for a public school environment, but nearly all of what is written here can be applied to a private school environment. However, in a private school environment you may not have as many rights to information nor as much sway to change as in a public school environment.

issue #1: energy use

Questions to Ask

- Has a professional energy audit been performed in the past five years?
- Where can I read the final report?
- What has the school done to improve upon problems or take recommendations found in the report?

Solutions to Advocate

- If no professional energy audit has been conducted in the last five years, advocate that one is performed and made publicly available.
- If the school can improve upon problems or act on recommendations in an energy audit report, work with the school to make those improvements financially feasible. Improvements can be instituted over time if needed.

ALLIANCE TO SAVE ENERGY >> (www.ase.org) This nonprofit coalition has a fabulous Green Schools Program to help your school save energy through the efforts of students, faculty, and staff. The program centers around energy efficiency and conservation and includes lesson plans for teachers.

AMERICAN SOCIETY OF HEATING, REFRIGERATING, AND AIR-CONDITIONING ENGINEERS (ASHRAE) >> (www.ashrae .org/freeaedg) This organization has published an energy-saving guide titled *Advanced Energy Design Guide for K–12 School Buildings* that speaks to school engineers but can be a useful resource for you to bring to the attention of your child's school. This guide also addresses the use of daylight lighting.

>> The energy-efficiency information and focus on Energy Star in the first three chapters of this book can also be a valuable resource to you in understanding what the available energy-saving options are that would apply to your child's school and what might be gleaned from an energy audit.

issue #2: food service

Questions to Ask

- Does the cafeteria have a published menu?
- Does the cafeteria or school district publish an ingredient list for food they serve? Does that ingredient list state any other details about the food, like whether it is from a sustainable source or is USDA Organic?
- How is the food being served? Are reusable dishes, trays, and utensils used, or is lots of trash being produced from one-time-use items? Do you use Styrofoam?
- What is in the vending machines? Are there any items with reduced packaging? Are any items USDA Organic or purchased from local companies?

- What is being sold à la carte? How is it being packaged?

Solutions to Advocate

- Most schools publish a cafeteria menu but offer no further details; you need to approach the school district for additional information. Still, even the school district might not know anything about the food they purchase beyond the bulk price. Since your tax dollars and child's health give you a right to this information, do not hesitate to push for answers. Ideally, you want the school to move toward purchasing USDA Organic and sustainable seafood and to make purchases from local suppliers to reduce transportation costs and pollution.

- In terms of serving items, the idea is to get your child's school to stop using any type of Styrofoam and reduce or completely eliminate nonreusable dishes, trays, and utensils unless they are biodegradable and/or compostable. Yes, it costs money to wash dishes, but the waste generated from disposables is a greater ill.

- Unfortunately, snack and beverage vending machine items produce a lot of waste because each item is separately packaged. Additionally, oftentimes there are fewer locally made or organic product options with which to stock vending machines. There are, however, multiple actions you can take. One is to ask that all vending machines be removed, but know that some schools might not respond well because fundraising may be tied to these machines or culturally it may not be acceptable. Or you could also work with the district and the school to reduce the waste generated by these machines by offering to research available waste-reduced products. Yet another option is to offer to research and recommend locally made and organic vending options. Additionally, you can look into reverse vending machines, which accept empty beverage containers and return money, prizes, or vouchers back to the user—now that's motivation!

- À la carte meal items are becoming increasingly popular in school cafeterias. And because à la carte is often run by outside vendors, your school or school district may ask that you contact the vendor for more information. The good news is that the school or school district has contracts with these vendors that will eventually expire. If you don't like what a vendor offers or how they're serving it, put pressure on the vendor to change or put pressure on the school to contract with a different, greener vendor.

COMMUNITY FOOD SECURITY COALITION (CFSC) >> (www.foodsecurity.org) Has information and organizational tools for you to start a farm-to-school program.

FARM TO SCHOOL >> (www.farmtoschool.org) This is a great resource if you want to get a farm-to-school program started in your child's school or school district.

NATIONAL SUSTAINABLE AGRICULTURE INFORMATION SERVICE >> (www.attra.ncat.org) Has a fabulous *Bringing Local Food to Local Institutions: A Resource Guide for Farm-to-Schools and Farm-to-Institutions Programs* guide available online.

TOMRA >> (www.tomra.com) This company has provided redemption programs for school fundraising and is willing to consider school recycling programs where the school is a central hub for community recycling.

YO NATURALS >> (www.yonaturals.com) Provider of vending machines with healthier foods, including organic products.

make your child a green lunch

One way to ensure that your child is eating a greener lunch is by preparing it yourself. Some tips:

- Use a reusable lunch bag—preferably one that is labeled PVC-free.
- Use reusable containers and utensils for food items, reducing the use of plastic baggies, juice boxes, and disposables as much as possible.
- Cool with a nontoxic ice pack.
- Provide healthier food—think organic whenever possible, with lots of fruits and vegetables.
- Resources to help you include www.wastefreelunches.org and www.laptoplunches.com.

issue #3: waste collection

Questions to Ask

- What is the school doing about sorting its waste? Does the school need any volunteer help during lunchtime to help kids sort lunch waste?
- Are there recycling bins next to trash cans throughout campus? Are there separate bins for food-only waste?
- Is the school composting food waste? If yes, then how is that compost being used?
- Is the school's maintenance department sorting its waste into trash (recyclable and nonrecyclable), green waste (from landscaping maintenance), and hazardous waste (from any cleaning or maintenance project)? Is the green waste being reused as mulch?
- What kind of trash liners does the school use?
- Are old textbooks recycled?
- Are used printer cartridges recycled?
- Are the children and staff educated on how to sort their trash?

Solutions to Advocate

- It costs almost nothing for your child's school to actively sort its waste if everyone is educated to do so. At the very least, separate containers for food items (which can be turned into compost), recyclables, and regular trash should be provided.

- Composting food waste is usually an issue of educating your school. When your child's school administration learns how important composting is and that compost can turn into free, nontoxic fertilizer and mulch for the school's campus (a big money saver!), the school will likely take action. But this also means that the students need to learn what goes into a compost receptacle and what doesn't (no meat, oil, or bones). Because lunchtime trash sorting can be challenging for kids to figure out and remember, the school may benefit from lunchtime parent volunteers who can help watch over and direct lunchtime waste sorting.
- For your child's health, to save the school money, and to improve the environment, your child's school maintenance group needs to sort its waste into the following categories: trash (recyclable and nonrecyclable), green waste (waste from landscaping that can be turned into free mulch for the campus), and hazardous waste. The hazardous waste absolutely needs to be turned into the district or city hazardous waste collection facility.
- Schools generate a lot of trash, so the little detail of the trash bin's liner is important, too. Traditional plastic liners are virtually nonbiodegradable. Push your child's school to buy either 100 percent biodegradable or 100 percent compostable liners and then follow the recommended procedures to compost or dispose of the bags.
- Even if the school implements green waste practices, if the students and staff don't make an effort to sort their waste, all will be for naught. This is why education and leadership support is so important. Encourage your child's school to make an annual (or more often, if the program is new or not doing well) effort to educate students and staff on sorting waste.

- Ask your child's school to initiate a garbageless school lunch program in which students are asked to only bring reusable food and drink containers.
- Review the disposal guidelines and resources in chapter 4 for additional ideas and information.

issue #4: cleaning

Questions to Ask

- How are dishes, utensils, tables and counters, and appliances cleaned in the kitchen and cafeteria?
- How are classrooms and floors cleaned?
- What kinds of cleaning supplies and chemicals are used?
- What kinds of vacuums are used?
- Are there hand dryers instead of hand towels in the bathrooms?

Solutions to Advocate

- The great news is that green cleaning your school is usually a matter of education on alternative options and moving to suppliers offering green alternatives. Just like at home, an audit can be made of all the cleaning supplies and equipment your child's school uses. From this audit, prepare a spreadsheet and track what should be traded for a greener option, what efforts are being made to find and purchase an alternative, and when a greener option is in use.
- Suppliers of greener products are usually sourced locally through janitorial supply companies (also known as distributors). This means that it will take some effort and coordination with these distributors to find greener suppliers with greener products and to determine the effectiveness of the products. Ask if suppliers or distributors are willing to let your school try samples before making big purchasing decisions; this will make your school much more willing to try greener cleaning.
- The bigger purchases made when changing machinery can either be a longer-term goal or, with fundraising, can be more quickly implemented. You want your school to use vacuums and other floor-cleaning equipment that have high-efficiency filters (like

HEPA filters) to capture microscopic elements, which could have adverse health effects on your child and on the school staff.

- You want your child's school to stop using cleaning products with hazardous chemicals. By studying the MSDS or ingredient label of any product, you can learn what ingredients, harmful or not, exist in any cleaning product. It is always better that a product has a MSDS available, because that means the company is making an effort to fully disclose potential hazards. A more complete explanation of cleaning products and green cleaning can be found in chapter 4, beginning on page 93.

- Hand dryers are more eco-friendly than paper towels. They not only save your school money on towel purchases but also consume less energy (because paper manufacturing uses more energy, especially since paper towels need to be replaced quite frequently) and virtually eliminate bathroom waste. You can easily make the case for a dryer by creating a budget that outlines what it would cost to install a hand dryer versus paying for hand towels.

EXCEL DRYER >> (www.exceldryer.com) The award-winning Xlerator hand dryer for public restrooms uses 80 percent less energy than traditional hand dryers, gives your school a 95 percent savings over using paper towels, and dries hands super fast.

RESPONSIBLE PURCHASING NETWORK >> (www.responsible purchasing.org) Has a comprehensive *Green Cleaning in Schools* guide available for purchase.

issue #5: supplies

Questions to Ask

- What kinds of electronics are being used?
- What kinds of paper are being purchased?
- What other office and textbook supplies are being purchased?

Solutions to Advocate

- Work with your school to help them take advantage of standby modes on computers and recommend that they purchase Energy Star or other power-saving electronics. If you are working with a group of parents to green your child's school, ask someone who has computer expertise to volunteer to help improve practices involving electronics. More ideas about this are found in chapter 3.
- As greener manufacturing takes hold, recommend that when electronic upgrades are needed, products should be purchased from manufacturers who use the least amount of energy and utilize the greenest resources and materials to make the product. Again, more info is found in chapter 3.
- Paper is preferably chlorine free and made from recycled sources. If paper is donated from parents, ask that they donate only recycled paper.
- Look for other office supplies and textbooks from greener distributors. Big box stores like Staples (www.staples.com) and Office Depot (www.officedepot.com) have on site supplies and online green catalogs.
- Communicate with your textbook suppliers and ask that textbooks be printed on recycled paper.

ACME UNITED CORPORATION >> (www.acmeunited.com) Under its Westcott brand, the company sells a Kleenearth line of trimmers and scissors that utilizes recycled plastic in its handles.

AMPAD (www.ampad.com) Has an Envirotec line of recycled office supplies made from 100 percent recycled and 100 percent postconsumer waste content, indicated with packages printed with green leaves (find out more about what these percentages mean in chapter 8).

CONSERVATREE (www.conservatree.com) A nonprofit organization that has lots of educational resources and databases for you to learn more about and source more eco-friendly paper.

DIXON TICONDEROGA (www.dixonusa.com) Sells a green pencil called the Ticonderoga EnviroStik.

FISKARS (www.fiskars.com) Sells an Envirogrip line of recycled scissors with handles made from 30 percent recycled plastic.

GREENOFFICESTORE.COM An online retailer of green office supplies.

OFFICE DEPOT (www.officedepot.com) Has a *Green Book* of office supplies and a list of eco-friendly products online at www .officedepot.com/buygreen.

PILOT (www.pilotbegreen.us) This company has a BeGreen line of pens and mechanical pencils that are not only refillable but also made from recycled content (with full disclosure on how much recycled content was used in the manufacturing process).

SANFORD (www.sanfordcorp.com) Has a line of nontoxic Earthwrite pencils that are made from reclaimed wood.

STAPLES (www.staples.com and www.staples.com/ecoeasy) Has many eco-friendly office supplies including thousands of products incorporating recycled content.

TREECYCLE (www.treecycle.com) Online catalog of many green office supplies, including recycled papers.

(continued)

ZEBRA >> (www.zebra-eco.com) Has a line of pencils, pens, and highlighters that are made from 70 percent postconsumer waste materials, like used car headlights, CDs, cell phones, and plastic bags.

issue #6: transportation

Questions to Ask

- What are the school and school district using for school bus transportation? Have they considered hybrid or alternative-fuel buses?
- Is the school encouraging children to walk or bike to school?
- Does the school have a bulletin board or forum where parents can connect with each other to form carpools?

Solutions to Advocate

- Encourage the use and purchase of school buses that use hybrid or alternative-fuel technologies such as propane. This will not only reduce emissions but also save the school money on fuel (which also means less taxes needed to fuel school transportation). Check with your state's environmental department to see if there are grants available for securing cleaner buses.
- If your child's school district doesn't offer transportation, make the case for a busing system. Imagine how this could improve the air quality of your community and how much pollution could be eliminated if all parents were relying on school transportation instead of driving their children to and from school. Although this would be a budget issue for a school district, you can also take your case to the city's government (such as a city council meeting) so that they understand just how much cleaner the air would be through busing—especially if they purchase hybrid buses. The city can then be your ally for putting pressure on the school district if necessary.
- If the district or school has a bus system, request that bus drivers, as well as parents waiting to pick up their children, do not idle outside the school.

- Work with your child's school to encourage children to walk and/or ride their bikes to school. If the children are young, then parents can be encouraged to walk or ride with them. By walking or riding a bike to school, children can improve their health, and this also means fewer cars on the roadway— improving air quality. If safety issues are a concern, such as lack of sidewalks and bike lanes, or traffic issues, then these are additional concerns that can be jointly discussed with your child's school and the municipality in which you live.

- You may have no other option but to drive your child to school because of the distance. In this case, the school should encourage parents to carpool. Perhaps there can be a binder at the front desk, a bulletin board, or on online forum for parents to connect with each other.

AIRWATCH NORTHWEST >> (www.airwatchnorthwest.org) Offers an online anti-idling tool kit for reducing emissions at your child's school.

BLUE BIRD CORPORATION >> (www.blue-bird.com) Sells propane and natural gas–powered school buses. The company's manufacturing process incorporates parts and materials made from recyclables.

IC BUS >> (www.icbus.com) Sells a hybrid bus that reduces particulate emissions by up to 90 percent, reduces greenhouse gas emissions by up to 40 percent, and improves fuel economy by up to 70 percent.

WALK TO SCHOOL >> (www.walktoschool.org) This is a fabulous site that motivates and provides information on how you can encourage your children to walk or ride a bike to school. An annual Walk to School Day happens every October, and you can plan school events around that date.

issue #7: heating and cooling

Questions to Ask

- How well insulated (doors, windows, general insulation) is my child's school?
- Are there deciduous trees surrounding the school that could help cool it down in the warmer months and let the sun shine in during the colder months?
- Is there any solar system in place?
- Does the school have a heat pump system?
- How much natural light is allowed into the school?
- Are there any ceiling fans in the school?
- What kind of heating or cooling unit(s) are being used? Is it Energy Star rated?

Solutions to Advocate

- The heating and cooling of your child's school matters not just because of your child's comfort but also because (1) you want to reduce your community's taxes by reducing your school's bills, (2) you want to reduce airborne emissions produced when your child's school uses heating and cooling appliances, and (3) you want to reduce the energy used by your school because then you benefit your community's environment. Many heating and cooling problems boil down to building and maintenance issues, which were often set into place when the building was built. With the exception of planting a few more trees, adding some ceiling fans, and doing a simple upgrade with film on windows, making significant changes to the school's heating and cooling system can be a major budget issue. As a result, first tackle the smaller, less-expensive items that can still make a difference. Then, work on the more expensive items over time by asking that they be included in a school or district's budget. You can help by researching the cost savings a school could have by installing updated, more energy-friendly systems—this can help make the case for money saving and keep interest in making an upgrade sooner.

issue #8: lighting

Questions to Ask

- What kinds of lighting are used in my child's school? Any CFLs or Energy Star fixtures?
- Where is natural light being taken advantage of?
- Are there any motion sensors installed?

Solutions to Advocate

- The best light for color rendering, health, and saving energy is light from the sun. Unfortunately, however, if a school is already built without many windows, you are limited in what can be done without incurring large expenses. However, one doable window-adding option is skylights, which are more easily implemented than conventional windows. Make sure that if your child's school is due for a remodel that more windows are added onto the remodel budget; you can help by researching how high-efficiency windows can save the school money on electricity and provide a healthier environment for the students and staff.
- Many schools have windows but unfortunately cover them with blinds that are kept shut all day, while the lights are turned on. A healthier and cost-saving approach would be to turn off the lights during the day and open the blinds to let the sun light the room. If heat through the windows is a problem, then inexpensive heat-blocking window film can easily be applied.
- Ask that lightbulbs be changed to energy-efficient and daylight-labeled options. You can get both the energy savings and the simulated daylight quality from both fluorescent and LED-type lighting. Request that aging light fixtures be changed to Energy Star–certified fixtures. This will add additional energy savings for the school.
- Encourage the school to install motion sensors on lights, as long as the lights will stay on long enough to not reduce the life of any fluorescent lightbulbs (usually about fifteen minutes is needed). Motion sensors can save the school money, as most people do not turn off lights in public places.

the benefits of daylight

There are numerous studies that show that natural light from the sun makes your child smarter and healthier. Research shows that children can be 20 percent faster on math tests and 26 percent faster on reading tests when they get regular sunlight. Only daylight lighting, when compared to other types of lighting, has shown a consistent relationship with improved learning, better behavior, less aggression, higher achievement, more teacher-student cooperation, healthier body growth, more energy and overall wellness, and greater ability to overcome hyperactivity and learning problems.

Additionally, it has been proven that there are lower rates of absence in daylight-lit classrooms, and those same classrooms had significantly less energy consumption, better ventilation, and less noise (not as many heating or cooling machines running, especially when better ventilation planning was integrated with daylight lighting). In fact, a school can save between 22 and 64 percent when replacing artificial light with natural light from the outside.

issue #9: water

Questions to Ask

- Are all water faucets installed with low-flow and/or aerating features?
- Are there any sensors on faucets?
- Have more native plants been installed in the landscaped areas?
- Is there any drip irrigation in place? Is there any kind of weather-tracking watering system in place?

Solutions to Advocate

- A school's water bill can be significantly reduced through better management of outdoor irrigation and indoor water use. And since water costs a lot of money in most places, your school district and school will likely support the idea of saving money.

- Recommend that all faucets be retrofitted with aerators. This is one of the less expensive water-saving updates. You can do research to show how much water and money the school can save through these aerator installations.
- Any remodeling or new building can benefit from sensor faucets that are also low-flow with aeration, to reduce the possibility of wasted water.
- You want green spaces for the kids, but you also want to conserve water. Encourage the school to employ xeriscape principles that use more native plants, which need less irrigation water. Encourage the installation of drip irrigation systems and sprinkler systems that waste less water and possibly function off of weather-tracking systems. Nearly all of these updates are money-saving ones. The school's outdoor maintenance manager should also be a part of any discussion. Chapters 2 and 5 have more information on water conservation and outdoor irrigation.

issue #10: landscaping

Questions to Ask

- What is being done to reduce or eliminate herbicide, traditional fertilizer, and pesticide use?
- Is the school mulching green waste and using it as nontoxic fertilizer?
- Is the school using a compost program to provide nontoxic fertilizing?
- What xeriscape steps are being taken to plant native trees and plants?
- Is there an emphasis on replacing asphalt with greenscape?

Solutions to Advocate

- Similar to green cleaning, you want to make a change from toxic herbicides, fertilizers, and pesticides to more environmentally friendly practices. Usually it is simply a matter of education for the school to reduce or eliminate these toxic chemicals.

- Once the school learns that it can produce its own fertilizer by composting and mulching, the cost savings alone can pay for a mulching mower and composting supplies—and probably even pay for a phased approach to xeriscape improvements (see chapter 5).
- Encourage your school to install more shrubs, trees, and climate-appropriate grass and ground cover and use water-efficient irrigation systems. Greenscape has been proven to improve attention span and brain focus among children, not to mention the relaxation it offers and the cooling effects, which leads to lower utility bills.

GREEN SHIELD CERTIFIED >> (www.greenshieldcertified.org) An independent nonprofit certification program that has a directory of effective, prevention-based pest control providers who also minimize the use of pesticides.

THE IPM INSTITUTE OF NORTH AMERICA >> (www .ipminstitute.org/school.htm) This nonprofit organization has an initiative to help your child's school reduce pesticides and, instead, practice integrated pest management (IPM). Your school can also become an IPM STAR Certified School. IPM focuses on reducing or eliminating conventional pesticides and instead concentrates efforts on prevention and more ecologically friendly ways of managing pests. IPM practices can also make your child's school environment safer.

schools unpave

Several schools across the nation are ripping out their concrete and asphalt and installing greenscape to benefit students, staff, and the local communities. The Los Angeles Unified School District is one large-scale example.

In renovating hundreds of existing campuses, there has been a move to bring in more greenery—adding green soccer fields, planting trees around buildings to help them cool off, finding places for small garden spots, and creating cooler outdoor reading areas with benches and trees. In Baltimore, seven city schools are removing asphalt and adding greenspace in conjunction with partial funding from the National Fish and Wildlife Foundation.

In both of these examples, the schools are becoming a more enjoyable place for learning and for play, and the community looks healthier and more inviting.

issue #11: access to outdoors

Questions to Ask

- Do children have outdoor recess time?
- Can children eat their lunch outdoors if the weather allows?
- Is there a school garden?
- Is there outdoor physical education?

Solutions to Advocate

- Unless your school is located in a wall-to-wall concrete environment or there are extreme outdoor temperatures, there is no reason why your kids can't be outdoors for recess, lunch, and physical education. Unfortunately, in recent years, many schools have cut outdoor time because of increased pressure for academic achievement and testing, decreased funding, or a fear of liability. Encourage a policy change at your school. Outdoor time for kids can help with restlessness, but it also can improve academic performance and boost health due to exposure to natural sunlight. Plus, when it comes to the environment, outdoor time helps children appreciate and love nature. Without this, children will lose touch with the earth and not have a feeling of stewardship for the planet.
- A school garden is a great project for children, as it's a hands-on way to learn about biology, science, and the world around us. It can even be sponsored by a local nursery or hardware store.

- Ask the school to remove some of its asphalt and replace it with greenscape. This can help reduce the surrounding air temperature around the school, as greenscape promotes coolness while hardscape soaks up heat and radiates it all day.
- Support nature education field trips, including environmental and nature-oriented science projects and trips.

kid-friendly habitat

If you are looking for resources to encourage your child's school to allow outdoor time, there's no better resource than the Schoolyard Habitats Program from the National Wildlife Federation (www.nwf.org/schoolyard). The program can assist your school in developing outdoor habitat areas that are meant to not only protect wildlife but also boost the educational opportunities of students, teachers, and the community at large. You can find training courses and curricula online, as well as support for finding funding.

a no-roof school

An interesting trend starting in Portland is the idea of outdoor schools. The Shining Star Waldorf School (www.shiningstarschool.com) in northeast Portland has partnered with the Tryon Life Community Farm and has an all-outdoor Mother Earth Kindergarten program that immerses the children in nature. The farm is sustainable, on seven acres, comes equipped with goats and chickens, and is right next door to 700 acres of public forestland. While the trend might be new in the United States, there are outdoor schools in Denmark, Norway, Sweden, and Finland.

how to start a school garden

Working with your child's school to set up a school garden requires several steps but is highly rewarding. School gardens not only expose your children to nature and the effort and care it takes to grow food and plants, but it also allows for outdoor time, science projects, and the eating of harvests. Here are some basic steps you can take to start a school garden:

1. Talk with the school principal about the idea and get school support.

2. Find an acceptable garden location on the school's property.

3. Assemble a support team—include parents with gardening/horticulture knowledge, maintenance personnel who can also assist with irrigation and composting, community sponsors to pay for or donate supplies, and your city and regional resources to help with education and promotion (city gardening expert, local extension office, and botanical garden). Oftentimes a local garden center is willing to be a sponsor. Additionally, Lowe's (www.lowes.com) has a Charitable and Educational Foundation that supports an Outdoor Classroom Grant Program that you can apply for to obtain supporting funds.

4. Talk with the teachers about what gardening programs would be useful teaching opportunities for their classrooms.

5. Create a plan of how the garden will be used, what will go into the garden, how it will be maintained, and what supplies are needed. Determine if the garden will only be seasonal or will also be maintained even when school is out of session.

6. Contact all school personnel, sponsors, parents, and other interested parties to let them know of the plan.

7. Begin collecting or purchasing supplies.

8. Implement the school garden.

9. Reap the rewards—eat harvested food for special lunches or salad bars at school, display flowers at a special event, present science learned at a school open house.

FOOD AND AGRICULTURAL ORGANIZATION OF THE UNITED NATIONS >> (www.fao.org) This organization has published online a helpful guide entitled *Setting Up and Running a School Garden.* Just type in the title of this guide in the Web site's search bar to find the link.

(continued)

NATIONAL GARDEN ASSOCIATION >> (www.kidsgarden.com)
This kid-oriented Web site of the NGA offers lots of help for parents, teachers, and volunteers setting up and maintaining a school garden.

issue #12: ventilation

Question to Ask

- How is the school getting fresh air into its rooms?

Solutions to Advocate

- Your child needs just as much fresh air at school as at home. Fresh air circulation can improve air quality and reduce the spread of germs, especially when there are a lot of people interacting with each other.
- As long as safety is not compromised, your school can improve fresh air flow by opening up windows and doors to let air circulate.
- Additionally, a fresh air ventilation system can also be installed into the central air system. More information about this is found in chapter 1.
- If children are periodically allowed to go outdoors this can supplement access to fresh air.

issue #13: construction

Question to Ask

- How green will any new construction be?

Solutions to Advocate

- If a new school is going to be built or if there will be any remodeling or additional construction at your current school, you have the right to know what will be constructed and how it will be accomplished. As a result, this is the perfect time to give input to your school and school district about constructing a green building from the ground up. There is more information about building and remodeling in chapter 3.

COLLABORATIVE FOR HIGH PERFORMANCE SCHOOLS >> (www.chps.net) Oversees a green building rating program for schools K–12.

Work Directly with Your School's Principal ✚

When it comes to ways of implementing the Green School Action Blueprint, working with your school's principal is one avenue. You'll want to set an appointment and prepare ahead. Here are some guidelines:

1. Be positive.
2. Come with a clearly outlined problem or issue.
3. Present possible solutions.
4. Be willing to work with the administration toward solving the problem, including volunteering some of your time, if possible.

Join a Parent-School Group ✚ ☼

Many schools have parent-school or parent-teacher groups that create an avenue for parents to discuss issues with the school that are important to them and their children. As long as the school and the group have a respectful and success-oriented relationship, it can be effective in making your child's school a positive place. Use the group to address your concerns about environmental issues and discuss the best ways to work with the school in developing improvements and change. Once you have gained support from others in the group and have a plan to move forward, the school or school district can be contacted in a thoughtful and positive way.

power in the pta

The Parent-Teacher Association (www.pta.org) is a good example of a national organization that helps to foster grassroots-level initiatives at your child's school; and the organization supports environmental initiatives as well, including nontoxic cleaning and reduction of air pollution and pesticides. There are also independent parent-teacher organizations that are run as nonprofit organizations and serve the same purpose at the local level as the PTA. In either case, these groups bring local parents together to improve the health, safety, and academics of their children at school and in the community.

Voice Your Interests in a School Board Meeting ✛ ☼

On your own or as a designated representative of a parent-teacher group, you can thoughtfully voice your green concerns at your school district's board meeting. Contact your school district to find out when the board meets and what their policy is for public comments. Public comments are better accepted when they include the following:

- A diplomatic tone.
- Well-thought-out and researched points—remember, budgetary concerns will be a sensitive issue, so if you can save money, this will help gain support.
- Recommended solutions.
- Supplementary information that has been prepared in advance to distribute to board members, which may include a summary of your comments and your recommendations, as well as solutions, details, and a sample budget.

Try to get the board to respond to your comments by asking them about their thoughts and reactions and what they feel might be the next step. Not only your comments but also the board's are recorded because it is a public meeting; because of this public record, proceedings are often published in your local newspaper, and this can help you to gain additional public support.

Serve on a School District Advisory Council ✚ ☼

Contact your school district office to see if they offer opportunities to serve on an advisory council. These are volunteer opportunities that help to advise the school board on such issues as finance, safety, transportation, and curriculum. Ask that a new council or committee be formed to advise on green issues.

Volunteer to Run a Green Program ✚ $

Schools are short on money, staff, and time, so volunteer—either alone or with the support of a group—to run a specific green program or initiative. Here are some ideas:

Develop a partnership: If you have a connection with an outside group or organization that is environmentally or nature minded, coordinate and be a liaison for a partnership between that organization and your child's school. For example, if you're a member of your local botanical garden, talk with the garden's staff about creating a pilot off-site garden at your child's school and a related field trip during the year. Your creativity and contacts can provide unlimited ideas.

Coordinate a special day or drive: Work with your school to coordinate a special recycling education day or an aluminum can drive.

THE CLEAN AIR CAMPAIGN >> (www.cleanaircampaign .com) This is a nonprofit organization based in Georgia that has lesson plans and tips for how to clean the air. If you live in the metro Atlanta area, there is also a school partnership program available.

(continued)

EARTHTEAM >> (www.earthteam.net) A network of business and education leaders, formed to help San Francisco Bay area schools and youth go green. There are lots of ideas on the Web site about how to green your school and community, and how to get youth to participate. And if you live in the San Francisco area, you can get involved.

THE FRUIT TREE PLANTING FOUNDATION >> (www.ftpf .com) This is a nonprofit charity dedicated to planting edible, fruitful trees and plants to help the environment and the people who enjoy them. They have a Fruit Tree 101 program that plants fruit trees in low-income schools.

GO GREEN INITIATIVE >> (www.gogreeninitiative.org) A school-specific go-green program that you can initiate at your child's school.

THE GREEN FLAG PROGRAM >> (www.greenflagschools.org) A program to help change environmental behaviors at your child's school to benefit your child's health and the environment.

ORGANIC CONSUMERS ASSOCIATION >> (www.organic consumers.org/afc) Has an Appetite for Change children's environmental health campaign that aims to get rid of pesticides at schools, transition school lunches toward healthier and more organic options, and teach children about sustainable agriculture (such as through a school garden).

ROOTS AND SHOOTS >> (www.rootsandshoots.org) Started by the legendary animal activist Jane Goodall, this youth club program helps you to start a group in your area that makes goals on helping your local environment and the community.

make your volunteering eco-worth it

Shelley Flint is a mom and the director of sustainability at San Domenico School in San Anselmo, California. She has these suggestions for parents who want to volunteer to help their child's school go more green:

- Research prices and rebates.
- Identify and run a fundraiser.
- Look for and apply for grants.
- Find local experts.
- Calculate savings.
- Write up recommendations.
- Research products and supplies.
- Identify local and organic food sources.
- Deliver recyclables to collection centers.
- Get quotes for projects from vendors.
- Help students sort waste at lunchtime.
- Work to help the school get off unwanted catalog lists.
- Offer to be the Eco-Mom of your child's classroom.

Talk to Your Local Retailer ✿ ☺

When you get your school supply list, drop a copy of it off at the places where you buy the supplies, along with a note to the store manager. Let him or her know that you would like more environmentally friendly options available for purchase, including:

- Reusable aluminum water bottles.
- Backpacks and lunchboxes that are PVC-free and are either made from recycled materials, organic cotton, hemp, or wool.
- Paper that is 100 percent recycled and chlorine free.
- Pencils that are certified by a responsible forest certification like the Forest Stewardship Council or made from recycled materials.

- Pens made from recycled materials that are also refillable.
- PVC-free scissors, rulers, and binders.
- Ask that all products made available be as nontoxic as possible.

THE CENTER FOR A NEW AMERICAN DREAM >> (www.new dream.org) and (www.shopbacktoschool.org) Has lots of back-to-school shopping tips and information with the focus on consuming less and being more environmentally friendly.

LIFESTYLE ACTION

promote a green community at large

what you need to know

I'll never forget the communications class I took in college in which the professor convinced me that one person can truly make a difference. He said that for every one person who writes to a TV station with a request, a complaint, or simple feedback, there are one hundred more people who felt the same way. His point was that savvy companies and organizations know this, so anyone who takes the time to write in is often taken seriously.

Since then, I have encountered even more dramatic statistics—that the one person represents one thousand people or more who felt the same way.

That one person who did something had a feeling of responsibility and acted to make a difference. When any of the Lifestyle Actions in this book become part of your routine at home, you will notice that you are making a difference.

The process in the community is the same, with one exception: Just as with your child's school and with your workplace, you can't tackle everything because it's not all doable at once. You have to make choices. How much time do you want to donate? How much money or other resources can you contribute? So take a look at the many ways you can influence, change, and then protect your community by action.

benefits
You and your family's health and safety will be protected, and your quality of life will be improved.

bringing up the issues
John Fentis, president of the Algalita Marine Research Foundation (www .algalita.org), strongly believes in consumer advocacy as an important tool for positive change. Fentis says, "A familiar theme from government is that it doesn't have the budget or funds for environmental cleanup. So, then it's really the citizens who must ensure their quality of life, maintain standards, and ask for enforcement of environmental laws."

If you have an environmental concern, Fentis recommends that you hop on a computer and make a list of take-action organizations that are concerned about the same issue you are. Contact one or more of those organizations and start a conversation with someone on their staff about what can be done.

"It's best to identify the boundaries of a problem and then talk about how to best communicate the problem to awaken the awareness of public officials. It's always better to come to the table and work toward a solution," says Fentis. This may mean, for example, that a PowerPoint presentation is prepared for a meeting with a public official or member of the media to easily explain the problem, who is adding to the problem, who is affected and how, and present recommended solutions.

Also, when you involve and educate the media on issues, you ensure that these issues will be brought to the public's attention, which in turn forces public officials and businesses to face problems that aren't being solved. A public official's ability to be reelected is put in jeopardy if he or she does not serve a constituency. And, "businesses can't hide behind lobbying and message design to deflect a problem and divert responsibility when they helped cause the problem," says Fentis.

how-to's

Vote Green ☺ ✚

With the environment becoming an increasingly pressing issue, most people running for public office (at any level) will state their positions on various environmental issues. Many of these folks have a Web site that breaks down issues and expands on statements, including environmental issues. Sometimes local political contenders hold public meetings where you can ask questions about their views, and incumbents often have a history of voting green or not green. Stay informed by reading your newspaper and joining environmental groups that will help you understand issues so that you can make informed political decisions. And if you find out a political candidate or public officeholder doesn't have a good environmental record, write a letter not only to that representative but also to the editor of your local paper to inform and influence others about this fact.

>> **Make your voice heard! Register to vote today.**

CLEAN WATER ACTION >> (www.cleanwateraction.org) Lists all the clean water–oriented legislation currently in process, both on the state and federal level, and what you can do to vote for or support cleaner water initiatives.

HEALING OUR WATERS—GREAT LAKES COALITION >> (www.healthylakes.org) Helps raise awareness of how your vote or publicly expressed opinion can help to clean up the Great Lakes.

THE LEAGUE OF CONSERVATION VOTERS >> (www.lcv.org) This organization makes available a scorecard of political leaders and their record on the environment. There is also a link to your state's league on the organization's home page. Both the federal

and state branches of the LCV can help you track other opportunities to vote in favor of the environment on both the national and
state levels.

SIERRA CLUB >> (www.sierraclub.org) Often lists environmental
voting records of federal house and senate leaders.

Lend a Hand ☺ ✚

Without volunteers, most community and nonprofit efforts would cease
to exist. There is simply not enough money to pay everyone whose help
is needed. Were it not for volunteer opportunities, many individuals
would find themselves disconnected from their communities.

Volunteering is all about time and passion, so you have to assess
how much time you have available and what you're passionate about.
You might only have enough time to help with a city or regional event
twice a year. Or perhaps you're in a situation where you can devote
enough time to run an event. Maybe you're willing to spend a vacation
volunteering (examples are in chapter 7), where the majority of your time
is spent either outside helping nature, conducting environmental research, or promoting findings of critical environmental information and
studies.

The best volunteer opportunities are those that you care about, because then it doesn't feel like work at all—just pure joy. This is why you not
only need the time available but also the passion. What do you feel passionate about? Clean beaches, waterways, and sustainable oceans?
Healthy forests? Gardening? Conducting research? Places you can go to
find these opportunities include your local aquarium, zoo, wildlife center,
state or local park department, botanical garden, child's school, local university, city volunteer center, city recycling center, think tank, take-action
group, or eco-tourism travel agent. Often there are also city, local newspaper, or school board advisory groups or committees to which you can apply to donate time on a community level; these groups allow you to have a
direct hand in recommending good environmental policy. You just have to

pick up the phone and ask if there are opportunities available or do some research on the Internet.

AMERICAN RIVERS >> (www.americanrivers.org) You can find river cleanups at this take-action group's Web site and volunteer your time.

ARBOR DAY FOUNDATION >> (www.arborday.org) Links to affiliate organizations that have tree-planting volunteer opportunities.

CLEAN OCEAN ACTION >> (www.cleanoceanaction.org) Offers volunteer opportunities to clean up beaches in the New Jersey and New York areas.

EARTH DAY NETWORK >> (www.earthday.net) This site lists environmental events that you can participate in not only for Earth Day but also throughout the year.

EARTH HOUR >> (www.earthhour.org) Every year there is a promotional earth hour when everyone across the globe is encouraged to turn off their lights to send a message about climate awareness. This Web site tells you more about how to get involved.

HEAL THE BAY >> (www.healthebay.org) If you live in or are traveling to California, you can get involved in the many clean-the-beach volunteer opportunities with this action organization.

KEEP AMERICA BEAUTIFUL >> (www.kab.org) An excellent organization that connects you with volunteer opportunities to improve your community's environment.

THE NATURE CONSERVANCY >> (www.nature.org) Volunteer opportunities in almost every state to help nature and the environment.

POINTS OF LIGHT AND HANDS ON NETWORK >> (www
.handsonnetwork.org) On this nonprofit's Web site, you can easily
search for environmental volunteer opportunities in your area.

SURFRIDER FOUNDATION >> (www.surfrider.org) Extensive
volunteer opportunities exist at this organization where you can
help to protect our oceans and beaches.

VOLUNTEER MATCH >> (www.volunteermatch.org) Matches up
volunteers with nonprofits and businesses with businesses' civic
activities.

Create Eco Programs ☺ ✚

If you have the time, passion, and leadership ability you can look into developing an environmental program in your community. The best programs are those that meet a real need and fill a gap as opposed to
duplicating someone else's efforts. Here are some ideas:

Work with your child's school to create a program and run it.
There are dozens of ideas in the school section earlier in this
chapter on how to donate your time.

Develop a donation program that not only meets a community
need but also cleans up waste that might otherwise be put in
a landfill. Work with a local business or businesses to sponsor
drop-off days and/or locations, generate publicity, and get
other volunteers to help you get the donated items to those
in need. Examples of community needs are gathering up
used eyeglasses, medical equipment, clothes, computers, or
paper.

Contact a local action organization, such as a branch of one of
the take-action organizations listed in the Resources section

of this book, beginning on page 304. Tell them you have an interest in volunteering and would love to spearhead a new program or be a replacement leader. Sometimes the organization will want to get to know you first, so you can make your entrance as a volunteer and then move to a leadership position after that.

Establish a community garden. If you like gardening, a fabulous project you can take on is a community garden. Community gardens bring people closer to nature and allow opportunities for growing your own food, helping the needy, preserving green space, cooling off neighborhoods (because there's no pavement in a community garden), and adding beauty.

AMERICAN COMMUNITY GARDENING ASSOCIATION >> (www.communitygarden.org) Excellent resource on how to start a community garden, as well as a database of community gardens all across the United States.

GREEN GUERILLAS >> (www.greenguerillas.org) An innovative grassroots organization in New York City that helps both New York and Brooklyn residents set up community gardens.

Express Your Opinion ☺ ✚

Don't underestimate the power of having your voice heard. Again, there are few who actually take the time to voice a concern, and there are many who feel the same way.

Here are some avenues for expressing your opinion:

- At a city council meeting—and bring some like-minded friends with you.
- At a zoning commission meeting—and, again, bring friends.

- At your homeowners' association meeting, where you might voice an opinion.
- By submitting comments to your local paper, either as a letter to the editor or a full-blown op-ed piece.
- On talk-radio programs where you can call in and express your opinion.
- Online comments, after an article or a blog posting.
- By writing a letter to government (city, state, federal) officials.
- By writing a letter to a company.

ENVIRONMENTAL DEFENSE >> (www.edf.org) This organization offers guidance on current environmental issues that you can write to your federal government officials and ask for action on.

NATURAL RESOURCES DEFENSE COUNCIL (www.nrdc.org/action) Also has take-action guidance for expressing your eco-friendly opinion in public.

When you express your opinion, you encourage thoughtful dialogue, present issues and solutions, and generate positive interest in change. Some of the issues you might address include:

Is there a sustainability plan for the city? You can see an example of a city's sustainability plan at www.sustainable-city.org; this is San Francisco's sustainability plan. There's another example of a sustainability plan in Northampton, Massachusetts, at www.northamptonma.gov. A sustainability plan means that your city is working to find a way to meet the needs of the present generation without sacrificing the needs and quality of life of future generations.

How can better public transportation be developed? You want less emissions, better access, and cost-effectiveness for mass transportation. Innovative ideas for public transportation, like a shared taxi service (for an example, you can read about www.texxi.com in London) or hybrid public transportation, can immediately reduce emissions and costs. Additionally, encourage your city to build and maintain sidewalks properly. You can also support bicycling and the installation of bicycle racks and paths. There are resources for addressing community bicycling problems at www .bicyclinginfo.org.

SAN FRANCISCO'S DEPARTMENT OF THE ENVIRONMENT >> (www.sfenvironment.org) You can click on "Our City's Policies" to find out information about the United Nations' Urban Environmental Accords which set environmental and sustainable standards to help your city create a sustainability plan. Cities from around the world have signed on to these accords to green their communities.

U.S. MAYORS CLIMATE PROTECTION AGREEMENT (www .usmayors.org/climateprotection) City mayors can sign on to this agreement, which gives targets and guidance in creating a sustainability and environmentally conscious plan.

>> By 2012, New York City wants to replace all its taxi cabs with hybrid vehicles.

What is being done with energy and water conservation? One innovative action you can take is to encourage your community to build and maintain smaller, community-oriented power plants instead of centralized, massive power plants that serve a whole region; centralized power plants are rarely as cost-effective as locally run plants and are not as versatile in integrating green energy options, like wind power. See chapters 1–3 and 7 for additional energy- and water-saving ideas.

Is the community addressing the need for people to live closer to work? It is better for the environment and for quality of life if people live and work in the same community. This environmental element is closely linked with economic-development and land-use plans, all of which your city's government and their agencies control.

cut your miles and improve your lifestyle

According to research done by think tank Urban Land Institute (www.uli .org), technology alone cannot reduce excessive greenhouse gases. As a result, people and cities must also change.

One change that the think tank recommends is that people reduce the number of miles they drive. According to the ULI, "Americans drive so much because we have given ourselves little alternative. For sixty years, we have built homes ever farther from workplaces, located schools far from the neighborhoods they serve, and isolated other destinations—such as shopping—from work and home." And one of the better ways, says the organization, is to create communities in which people work, live, shop, and play—without having to drive a long distance; or maybe even walk to work. Redevelopment and infill development (filling in vacant land instead of building out farther away from the city and destroying habitats) would help create this type of mixed-use, denser living.

How is green space being preserved? Policies need to be set that preserve a minimum percentage (as much as possible because virgin habitats are rapidly disappearing) of green space and animal habitats *within* an urban setting, including sufficient trees for birds and other small animals. Outside of urban areas, even more green space and habitats need to be permanently preserved. Restoration of habitats and green space may also be an issue. You can also look at the condition and quantity of your local and regional parks. And you can encourage the building of wildlife crossings on freeways and highways to enhance and protect wildlife diversity and their access to food and water—not to mention a safety impact of not hitting and killing these animals.

>> According to the nonprofit group American Forests (www .americanforests.org), since 1972 American cities have lost more than a quarter of their tree canopies. This happens as urban areas continue to grow and destroy once-virgin habitat.

How can air and water pollution be reduced and more closely regulated? Support efforts to mandate that vehicle emissions be reduced by even greater percentages. Ask for transparency from companies as to what they are expelling into the air and water. Look for ways to encourage your community to recycle wastewater as reclaimed water for irrigation and other public uses— this helps avoid the need to build new dams or to over-tap underground aquifers. Ask that your city publish an annual water quality report. If part of your community is composed of rural farming, see what can be done about requiring less pesticide use (this will protect your water and help wildlife such as bees).

TOX TOWN >> (www.toxtown.nlm.nih.gov) This interactive Web site of the U.S. National Library of Medicine helps you identify environmental health concerns in your city, town, port, or on your farm.

How is the local landfill being managed? Poorly managed landfills and landfills near or on areas where people live can have unwanted health and environmental effects due to the release of toxic gases and seepage into groundwater. And incinerators can be hugely air polluting. Require your city to make public a nonbiased, third-party periodic report about the status of any recommendations for your landfill.

What is being done to encourage a zero-waste goal in your community? Zero waste means you change habits and processes to reach a goal of no waste in your community—or at least get very close. Encourage your city's officials to work with its residents, businesses, and municipal services to move toward a zero-waste goal. The first step in moving toward zero waste is to reduce consumption. The second step is to recycle and compost what you cannot eliminate. This means the city would a have a substantial reduction in trash, yard clippings, and paper. Composting would be heavily promoted. Certain kinds of plastics, like polystyrene foam (Styrofoam), could also be banned, while biodegradable plastics would be encouraged. And recycling efforts and goals could be ramped up for residents, businesses, and city departments. City ordinances or state laws can regulate waste, plastics, recycling, and other conservation and waste issues. When cities and states make changes that are better for the environment, providers of products follow suit by finding ways to still sell you their wares but still meet new environmental guidelines. As reported at a zero waste forum in May 2008, examples of large businesses who have already reached a greater than 90 percent zero-waste goal by designing waste out of their business processes are Apple Computers, Seiko Epson Corporation, Hewlett-Packard, Toyota, Xerox Corporation, IKEA, Ricoh Electronics, Pillsbury (a company of General Mills), the San Diego Wild Animal Park, and Safeway grocery stores.

ECO-CYCLE >> (www.ecocycle.org) Nonprofit recycler with many resources and ideas on zero waste and recycling.

GARY LISS & ASSOCIATES >> (www.garyliss.com) Unique consulting services for communities and businesses to help them draft and implement zero-waste plans and resource recovery.

(continued)

THE GRASSROOTS RECYCLING NETWORK (www.grrn.org) Educational and resource site for learning more about zero waste and how you can work with your community to create zero-waste goals.

THE ZERO WASTE ALLIANCE (www.zerowaste.org) A nonprofit organization dedicated to educating, assisting, and being a resource for zero-waste goals of communities and organizations.

ZERO WASTE INTERNATIONAL ALLIANCE (www.zwia.org) An organization dedicated to zero waste. Individuals, businesses, organizations, and governments can belong to this organization and pledge to adhere to the Alliance's zero-waste principles.

what it will take to get to zero waste

Speaking on how to obtain a zero-waste society, Eric Lombardi, executive director of Eco-Cycle (www.ecocycle.org) in Boulder, Colorado, says, "A revolution in thinking is required . . . the global economy was [once] built upon the bodies of slave labor . . . the current global economic engine for growth is built upon the destruction of our natural world. Slavery didn't end because of economic pressures."

Lombardi's point is that citizens must take it upon themselves to advocate that laws be changed that require companies to be more environmentally friendly. He believes this is the only way there will be a substantial change in making companies and their products cleaner, and he encourages citizens to create a Community Zero Waste Task Force. Involve local leaders who will support you, and use the media to your advantage.

a landfill the size of africa

Out in the middle of the Pacific Ocean, north of the Hawaiian Islands, is what is called the North Central Pacific Gyre. A gyre is a swirling vortex of water. This is an area of high pressure and clockwise rotating currents. If you took a satellite view of this area of the world, it would only show you clear blue waters. But the truth is that caught in this revolving flow is a floating garbage dump of mostly . . . plastic. Plastic debris that won't escape those currents unless all of us who let it drain into the sea are able to take it out—an enormously costly proposition.

The plastic floats somewhere between the surface and a couple of feet below—in bits and pieces, but never degrading. Fish and birds mistake the plastic for food, filling their insides with not only a toxic mess but also making it impossible to eat any real food because the plastic does not digest. The Algalita organization (www.algalita.org) has been researching this problem and many other environmental problems related to plastic waste and is an indispensable resource for you in understanding how you can help stem the tide of plastics and their waste in your community and with manufacturers.

Additionally, on Algalita's Web site research pages, they also have a life-changing video of a necropsy (postmortem examination) of a fledgling Laysan Albatross, which shows you just how much plastic is being consumed by wildlife.

How strong are the municipality's recycling efforts? Are separate recycling bins being provided for residents? Are residents educated on what they can recycle? Are recycling receptacles provided in public places like shopping centers, airports, stores, and government buildings? Is the city supporting a composting education program and free or discounted composting bins? What can the city do to require that residents and businesses recycle more?

What can be done to ban more toxic chemicals from products and their manufacturing processes? Working with take-action organizations is the best way to make this happen. They can assist you in meeting with public officials, explaining the problem and who it affects, and determining what solutions are possible. By informing your public officials and the media about the problem, you can help get laws passed that ban toxic products and put caps on manufacturing emissions and waste.

Join Green Action Groups ☺ ✚ $–$$

If there is an action group that you strongly support (see a list of several take-action groups in the Resources section of this book), consider joining. As a member of one of these groups, you will be better informed thanks to resources like e-mail or hard-copy publications, and your participation will help keep the organization's efforts afloat.

Donate to Improve the Environment ☺ ✚ $–$$$$

If you have the money to spare, you might consider donating your greenbacks to your favorite environmental organization. Beyond money, if you have land to donate, consider securing this space's future forever by donating it to preservation of habitat efforts. Donations can really make a difference in advancing an organization's mission and campaigns, and sometimes you can earmark donations to be used for specific initiatives. Finally, most donations to nonprofit organizations are tax deductible.

CHARITY NAVIGATOR >> (www.charitynavigator.org) This indispensable organization rates charities and nonprofits. You can use the rating to determine how effectively an organization you are interested in is run. You want to send your money to an organization that is fiscally responsible and financially healthy. Their Web site also has a search feature that lets you find four star-rated environmental groups.

THE WILDLIFE LAND TRUST >> (www.wlt.org) If you own land (small or large, urban or rural) that could be left to wildlife or preservation of habitat, this organization helps you permanently preserve and oversee your land through your land donation. You can also volunteer to monitor donated lands.

Invest Green ☺ ✚ $–$$$$

Investing green means putting your money at the source—with companies who are doing better for the earth, for your health, and for your safety. The easiest way to invest green is to ask your financial advisor to research green funds and socially responsible companies. The DIY approach is to search company reports to see if an organization discloses their climate-change risks and sustainability outlook. Another great way to express your opinion is to contact the Securities and Exchange Commission and encourage them to require that public companies disclose such information. If you are an entrepreneur and have enough cash to be a partner in, buy, or create a green business, this is another great investment option.

Run for Office ☺ ✚ $$$$

This is only for the determined and able, but running for office—and winning—puts you in an enviable position: You're able to exert a tremendous influence through decision-making power to turn the tide toward a sustainable future. As a mother, you know better than most the full impact of society's good and bad, and you feel passionate about preserving your children's future. Running for office usually starts with a grassroots effort, and the more well connected you are, the easier it will be for you to compose a team who will support you and find donors to fund your campaign. The good news is that if you are strongly pro environment, you can look for support from eco-friendly organizations and businesses and their contacts.

AIR QUALITY

Air Now (www.airnow.gov) • A U.S. government agency Web site that gives you current and forecasted information on the air quality in your area.

ALTERNATIVE HEALTH CARE

The American Association of Naturopathic Physicians (www.naturopathic.org) • Has a searchable database of naturopathic physicians.

American Chiropractic Association (www.amerchiro.org) • Offers chiropractic information and a chiropractor search feature.

The Council for Homeopathic Certification (www.homeopathicdirectory.com) • Provides a directory of certified homeopathic professionals.

National Center for Complementary and Alternative Medicine (www.nccam.nih.gov) • A government Web site for information on preventive and complementary care.

National Center for Homeopathy (www.nationalcenterforhomeopathy.org) • Has study groups across the United States to learn more about homeopathy.

National Certification Commission for Acupuncture and Oriental Medicine (www.nccaom.org) • Has information on acupuncture and eastern medicine.

BUILDING AND REMODELING

Cradle to Cradle (www.c2ccertified.com) • This is a certification used on a wide variety of products that are sustainable, reusable, and recyclable.

Efficient Windows Collaborative (www.efficientwindows.org) • This organization has a terrific Web site that provides resources for upgrading to energy-efficient windows in your home.

Energy and Environmental Building Association (www.eeba.org) • Green building information.

Energy Savers (www.energysavers.gov) • Lots of tips and information on green building and energy savings.

Environmental Stewardship Program seal (www.greencabinetsource.org) • Certification for greener cabinetry administered by the Kitchen Cabinet Manufacturers Association.

GreenGuard (www.greenguard.org) • Certification for indoor products with low emissions and has a searchable database for flooring, doors, insulation, paints, and wall finishes.

The Green House (www.nbm.org) • Look under 2007 exhibitions for the Green House at this Web site of the National Building Museum. There are tons of ideas and product listings from this exhibit of sustainable living and architecture.

Hansen Living (www.hansenliving.com) • Makes eco-friendly, long-lasting kitchens and bathrooms out of wood from responsibly managed forests.

LEED certification (www.usgbc.org) • Green building and remodeling third-party certification administered by the U.S. Green Building Council.

National Fenestration Rating Council (www.nfrc.org) • Rates and compares the energy and performance of windows, doors, and skylights. This Web site also has a certified product directory.

CLEANING

CleanerSolutions Database (www.cleanersolutions.org) • Database of cleaning products. You can sort by what you want to clean and product safety scores.

Consumer Product Safety Commission (www.cpsc.gov) • U.S. agency responsible for protecting consumers from serious injury or death from more than 15,000 types of products; lists recalls and product safety news.

Design for the Environment (DfE) (www.epa.gov/oppt/dfe) • Labeling program by the EPA that certifies products as safer for humans and better for the environment.

EcoLogo (www.ecologo.org) • Seal of green certification for North American (United States and Canada) products.

Green Seal (www.greenseal.org) • Independent green certifier of household products, building materials, and lodging.

National Institutes of Health's Household Products Database (http://household products.nlm.nih.gov) • Online database of household products, their ingredients, and their MSDSs.

COSMETICS

Aveda (www.aveda.com) • The company and its personal care products are dedicated to product safety, responsible ingredient sourcing, utilizing more natural and organic ingredients, reducing packaging and using recycled materials in its packaging, and powering its operations with renewable energy.

Cosmetic Safety Database (www.cosmeticsdatabase.com) • You can type cosmetics by name into the search engine and learn about any chemical hazards. This Web site also has a parents' buying guide for children's personal care products.

Green by Nature (www.greenbynaturebeauty.com) • Personal care products that are 100 percent paraben, DEA, and sulfate free.

Leaping Bunny (www.leapingbunny.org) • Certifies cruelty-free products.

Physicians Formula (www.organicwearmakeup.com) • Sells an Organic Wear line of cosmetics that is 100 percent free of harsh chemicals and synthetic preservatives and colors, 100 percent cruelty free, 100 percent free of parabens and GMOs, uses up to 93 percent less plastic for some of its containers, and integrates U.S.-certified organic ingredients into this product's line.

ENERGY

Alliance to Save Energy (www.ase.org) • You can find many tips, resources, and miniguides on the Web site for this consumer- and community-friendly organization.

American Council for an Energy-Efficient Economy (www.aceee.org) • Great tips and links for green living.

Consortium for Energy Efficiency (www.cee1.org) • Online databases that categorize residential products in tiers of energy efficiency.

Database of State Incentives for Renewable Energy (www.dsireusa.org) • State-by-state clickable database of incentives and rebates for going green.

Electronic Product Environmental Assessment Tool (www.epeat.net) • Rates computers, laptops, and monitors based on their environmental impact.

Energy Star (Canada) (http://oee.nrcan.gc.ca or www.oee.nrcan.gc.ca/energystar/english/consumers/index.cfm) • Additional information on water efficiency of dishwashers that is not currently listed in the Energy Star program in the United States.

Energy Star (U.S.) (www.energystar.gov) • Lots of information about saving energy and Energy Star–rated products.

Florida Solar Energy Center (www.floridaenergycenter.org) • Includes research on solar energy systems (photovoltaics or PV technology) as well as a list of certified PV systems.

Geothermal Heat Pump Consortium (www.geoexchange.us) • Excellent resource on how geothermal heat pumps work. Also lists geothermal heat pump manufacturers.

The Green Power Network (www.eere.energy.gov/greenpower) • A useful site from the Department of Energy that helps you find green power options where you live.

Lighting Research Center (www.lrc.rpi.edu) • A university-based research and educational organization devoted to lighting.

My Green Electronics (www.mygreenelectronics.com) • How to recycle and reuse electronics, as well as find greener new electronic options. A product directory is available on the site.

National Lighting Bureau (www.nlb.org) • Nonprofit lighting industry advocate for high-benefit (energy-efficient) lighting.

Professional Awning Manufacturing Association (www.awningstoday.com) • Information and ideas on how awnings can reduce your energy costs and improve your property value.

Solar Energy Industries Association (www.seia.org) • Information about solar power and links to information about state and federal incentives/rebates.

Solar Gard (www.solargard.com) • Heat control window film manufacturer.

Tankless Water Heater Guide (www.tanklesswaterheaterguide.com) • Details the specifics on how tankless water heaters work.

U.S. Department of Energy (www.energy.gov) • A wonderful Web site with a lot of unbiased information about saving energy. There is also a DOE division of Energy Efficiency and Renewable Energy (www.eere.energy.gov) that has additional resources specific to green living.

FOOD

The Association of Junior Leagues International (www.ajli.org) • Has a fun Kids in the Kitchen program that gets parents and kids involved in cooking healthy at home.

Center for Food Safety and Applied Nutrition (www.cfsan.fda.gov) • Information on how to read the nutrition facts label.

Certified Humane (www.certifiedhumane.com) • A third-party certification to ensure animals raised for food are treated humanely and offered a nutritious diet.

Co-op Directory Service (www.coopdirectory.com) • An easy-to-use directory of co-ops.

The Cornucopia Institute (www.cornucopia.org) • Has a helpful online dairy report and scorecard to determine the integrity of your organic milk.

Eat Local America (www.eatlocalamerica.coop) • Information about local co-ops and farmers.

Environmental Working Group (www.foodnews.org) • Offers a useful Pesticides in Produce guide.

Food Alliance Certified (www.foodalliance.org) • Certifies sustainable agriculture.

Green Restaurant Association (www.dinegreen.com) • This nonprofit organization has an online guide to green-certified restaurants.

Local Harvest (www.localharvest.org) • A database of farmers' markets, community supported agriculture farm programs (CSAs), and other local food initiatives.

Marine Stewardship Council label (www.msc.org) • Certifying label of fish products that are well managed and not overfished.

My Pyramid (www.mypyramid.gov) • U.S. government's Web site to teach you about food and eating right.

National Organic Program (www.ams.usda.gov/NOP) • Site for information and regulation of the USDA Organic label.

Sustainable Table (www.sustainabletable.org) • Illustrates problems with our current food supply and offers solutions and alternatives.

U.S. Department of Agriculture's Agricultural Marketing Service (www.ams.usda.gov) • Has a farmers' market search page and information about the USDA Organic label.

GARDENING

American Community Gardening Association (www.communitygarden.org) • Excellent resource on how to start a community garden, as well as a database of community gardens all across the United States.

Association of Specialty Cut Flower Growers (www.ascfg.org) • Online, state-by-state flower buyers guide.

Ball Food Storage (www.freshpreserving.com) • Information on preserving your home produce.

Beyond Pesticides (www.beyondpesticides.org) • Nonprofit organization that provides information on pesticides and their alternatives.

Greenscapes program (www.epa.gov/greenscapes) • A government certification program that offers environmentally friendly solutions for landscaping.

Green Shield Certified (www.greenshieldcertified.org) • An independent, nonprofit certification program that has a directory of pest control providers who minimize the use of pesticides.

National Garden Association (www.garden.org) • A nonprofit organization that promotes gardening. The organization also maintains a sister Web site dedicated to encouraging children and families to garden at www.kidsgardening.org.

Natural Resources Conservation Service (www.nrcs.usda.gov) • Has a searchable database of thousands of plant species in the United States.

Organic Gardening (www.organicgardening.com) • A magazine devoted to organic gardening.

U.S. Department of Agriculture's Cooperative Extension Office (www.csrees.usda .gov/Extension) • Experts can help teach you how to garden and what to garden in your area and climate during the various seasons; there are local extension offices not far from most communities across the United States.

Veriflora (www.veriflora.com) • Third-party certification for sustainable flowers.

GENERAL RESOURCES

Biodegradable Products Institute (www.bpiworld.org) • Offers an approved list of plastic products that will biodegrade and compost.

Bird-Friendly seal (www.si.edu/smbc) • Shade-grown certification by the Smithsonian Migratory Bird Center to help protect migratory birds and their habitats.

Buy Less Crap (www.buylesscrap.com) • List of charitable causes you can donate to.

Care 2 Make A Difference (www.care2.com) • Online community of people interested in the care of our environment.

The Center for a New American Dream (www.newdream.org) • An excellent resource on how to be a conscious consumer, plus lots of eco-friendly tips and links.

Charity Navigator (www.charitynavigator.org) • This organization rates charities and nonprofits.

Earth 911 (www.earth911.org) • Portal for environmentally focused resources. The site also has a helpful tool to locate recycling and hazardous waste centers for your area.

Eartheasy (www.eartheasy.com) • Sustainable living ideas.

EnviroLink (www.envirolink.org) • A resource for many green living topics.

Enviromom.com (www.enviromom.com) • A terrific site for parents to get ideas from one another on a myriad of green topics.

Family.com (www.family.com) • This Disney-owned Web site has a green living section where parents share eco ideas.

Goodwill (www.goodwill.org) • Organization that accepts household and clothing donations.

Greener Choices (www.greenerchoices.org) • Archived *Consumer Reports* articles on green living-oriented appliances, cars, electronics, foods, and beverages.

GreenHomeGuide (www.greenhomeguide.com) • General resource of tips and information on green living.

Low Impact Living (www.lowimpactliving.com) • Offers hundreds of suggestions for going green.

Mothers & More (www.mothersandmore.org) • Local chapters of mothers who want to connect with other mothers. A great place to meet and team up with fellow green moms.

Salvation Army (www.salvationarmyusa.org) • Nonprofit that accepts household and clothing donations.

San Francisco's Department of the Environment (www.sfenvironment.org) • You can click on "Our City's Policies" to find out information about the United Nations' Urban Environmental Accords, which set environmental and sustainable standards to help your city create a sustainability plan. Cities from around the world have signed on to these accords to green their communities.

Transfair USA (www.transfairusa.org) • Independent, third-party certifier of fair trade products in the United States.

TreeHugger.com (www.treehugger.com) • A plethora of green living tips, news, product information, public forums, and blogs.

Tufts Climate Initiative (www.tufts.edu/tci) • Focuses on ways to reduce climate changes, including CO_2 reductions.

U.S. Environmental Protection Agency (www.epa.gov) • Overall resource on hundreds of environmental topics. A subsection of this Web site gives climate change history, current events, and future projections, as well as tips, at www.epa.gov/climatechange. The WaterSense section is found at www.epa.gov/watersense.

U.S. Mayors Climate Protection Agreement (www.usmayors.org/climateprotection) • City mayors can sign on to this agreement, which gives targets and guidance in creating a sustainability and environmentally conscious plan.

The Wildlife Land Trust (www.wlt.org) • This organization helps you permanently preserve and oversee your land through your donation. You can also volunteer to monitor donated lands.

Worldwatch Institute (www.worldwatch.org) • An organization that creates reports and publications related to environmental issues.

GREEN RETAILERS, MANUFACTURERS, AND SERVICE PROVIDERS

3M (www.3m.com) • Clear-window, energy-saving window film—dealer installed only.

AFM Safecoat (www.afmsafecoat.com) • Zero-VOC paints and sealers.

American Air Filter (www.americanairfilter.com) • Nonfiberglass disposable air filters.

American Standard (www.americanstandard-us.com) • Low-flow and dual-flush technology toilets and showerheads with high-efficiency WaterSense labeling.

Ampad (www.ampad.com) • Has an Envirotec line of recycled office supplies made from 100 percent recycled and 100 percent postconsumer content, indicated with packages printed with green leaves.

Amsoil (www.amsoil.com) • Synthetic automobile oil made from renewable resources.

Aramark (www.aramark.com) • Environmentally focused food service company.

Arm & Hammer (www.armhammer.com) • Baking soda and washing soda, as well as HEPA vacuum filters at www.armhammervac.com.

Aveda (www.aveda.com) • This cosmetics and hair care company has green, sustainability, and fair trade at the center of its business.

Avis (www.avis.com) • The car rental company is increasing its fleet of hybrid vehicles, along with a large portion of higher-fuel-efficiency vehicles.

Bamboosa (www.bamboosa.com) • Sells bamboo clothing and accessories, and has information about bamboo on its Web site.

Benjamin Moore & Company (www.benjaminmoore.com) • Has an Eco Spec line of paints that is lower in odor and low-VOC.

Beyond Learning (www.beyond-learning.com) • Kids' learning games printed with soy ink on recycled paper.

BioBay (www.biobayusa.com) • Compostable and biodegradable trash bags, shopping bags, and composting systems.

Biokleen (www.biokleenhome.com) • Biodegradable, concentrated, and nontoxic cleaning products.

Bissell (www.bissell.com) • Has an easy-to-use steam mop and several different types of HEPA-filtered vacuums.

Bite Blocker (www.biteblocker.com) • DEET-free insect repellent.

BoAir (www.boair.com) • Distributor of BoAir high-quality reusable electrostatic air filters for your central air system that are backed by a ten-year warranty.

The Body Shop (www.thebodyshop.com) • The company has a strict policy against animal testing on its ingredients and products, and also supports fair trade.

Bon Appétit Management Company (www.bamco.com) • Sustainable and responsible food service company.

Born Free (www.newbornfree.com) • Nontoxic baby bottles, nipples, and drinking cups.

Bosch (www.boschappliances.com) • High-quality appliances with long-term commitment to rating all of its appliances with the Energy Star certification—for cooking, laundry, and dish washing.

BP Solar (www.bpsolar.us) • Sells solar solutions for homes, businesses, and builders. A solar savings calculator is found on their site.

Brita (www.brita.com) • At-home water filtration by refrigerator filter, pitcher, or faucet mount.

Broan (www.broan.com) • Quality, Energy Star–rated home ventilation systems.

Burt's Bees (www.burtsbees.com) • Natural-ingredient personal care products.

California Organic Flowers (www.californiaorganicflowers.com) • USDA Organic flowers.

Carrier (www.carrier.com) • Complete line of energy-efficient heat pumps, ventilation, and air-conditioning products.

ChicoBag (www.chicobag.com) • Reusable shopping bags.

Chipotle Mexican Grill (www.chipotle.com) • Restaurant chain focused on sustainable and healthy food offerings.

Citra-Solv (www.citra-solv.com) • Cleaning products that are from naturally derived sources and renewable resources, along with full ingredient disclosure.

Climatemaster (www.climatemaster.com) • Geothermal heat pumps.

Crane Plumbing (www.craneplumbing.com) • High-efficiency WaterSense-certified toilets, including dual-flush version.

Dell (www.dell.com) • Comprehensive environmental initiatives for its electronics and computers, such as phasing out toxic substances from their products, adding in energy-efficiency features, and free recycling.

Delta (www.deltafaucet.com) • Water-efficient showerheads and faucets.

Derma E (www.dermae.com) • Cruelty-free personal care products made with eco-friendly ingredients in 100 percent recyclable packaging.

Diamond Organics (www.diamondorganics.com) • Organic foods and flowers.

Dirt Devil (www.dirtdevil.com) • Sells HEPA vacuums.

Dr. Benson's Natural Mix (www.drbensonsmix.com) • Natural fertilizer with no salts that is also safe for your garden produce.

Dropps (www.dropps.com) • Super-concentrated, eco-friendly laundry detergent that does not harm your clothes, your health, or the environment. Dropps also reduces waste by selling the product without a bottle or cap to recycle—the product comes in dissolvable packs.

Duracell (www.duracell.com) • Offers rechargeable batteries.

Earth Lighting (www.goodearthlighting.com) • Energy Star–rated lighting fixtures.

The Earth Machine (www.earthmachine.com) • Easy outdoor composter system that is often provided by local governments for free to residents. It is also available through vendors such as www.composters.com. The Earth Machine's Web site has lots of simple info on how to compost.

Earthshell (www.earthshellnow.com) • 100 percent biodegradable plates and bowls made from corn, potatoes, and limestone.

Eco-Products (www.ecoproducts.com) • Eco-friendly, sustainable, and nontoxic food service, janitorial, and household supplies.

Ecover (www.ecover.com) • Full line of eco-friendly household cleaning products that list ingredients.

Electrolux (www.electrolux.com) • Appliances and vacuums with eco-friendly and energy-saving features.

Element Hotels (www.elementhotels.com) • This hotel chain is dedicated to eco-friendly practices.

EM America (www.emamerica.com) • Has a product that can accelerate the composting process and help control odor.

Energizer (www.energizer.com) • Sells rechargeable batteries and chargers.

Enterprise Rent-A-Car (www.enterprise.com) • Has a growing fleet of hybrid vehicles for rent, along with higher-fuel-efficiency vehicles.

Epson (www.epson.com) • Sells Energy Star–rated electronics. The company has an extensive recycling program, a goal of zero waste in its manufacturing (which also saves resources), programs to reduce packaging, and a control initiative to eliminate harmful substances and replace them with safer alternatives.

ETWater (www.etwater.com) • Smart-controller system uses weather data to automate and optimize your landscape watering schedules.

Evite (www.evite.com) • A free service for sending electronic party invitations.

Excel Dryer (www.exceldryer.com) • Has an award-winning Xlerator hand dryer for public restrooms that uses 80 percent less energy than traditional hand dryers and dries your hands super fast.

EZ-FLO (www.ezfloinjection.com) • Microdose fertilizer system done through your irrigation or sprinklers that results in much less fertilizer and water used and healthy plants.

FedEx (www.fedex.com) • Has a ground shipping option, as well as reusable envelopes.

Feit Electric (www.feitelectric.com) • Has a variety of lightbulbs, including antibug and low-mercury compact fluorescents.

FHP Manufacturing (www.fhp-mfg.com) • Geothermal and water-source heat pumps.

FindCO2.com (www.findco2.com) • This Web site helps you find a CO_2 dry cleaning store near you.

Fiskars (www.fiskars.com) • Sells an Envirogrip line of scissors with handles made from 30 percent postconsumer waste plastic.

FLOR (www.florisgreen.com) • Sells low-VOC and formaldehyde-free carpet tiles. The company also helps its customers recycle its carpets—FLOR arranges for the carpet to be picked up, returned, and recycled at no cost to you.

Ford (www.ford.com) • Sells hybrid vehicles under the Ford and Mercury brands.

Gaiam (www.gaiam.com) • Environmentally friendly products.

gDiapers (www.gdiapers.com) • Has flushable and/or compostable inserts and a fitted cloth diaper.

GE (www.ge.com) • Full range of energy-efficient appliances and lighting.

Giant (www.giant-bicycles.com) • Extensive line of bikes for all needs, along with a Suede Coasting bike that is great relaxing travel for a mom; also has a hybrid electric bike that can take you up to seventy-five miles per charge. Specific bike info for women can be found at www.giantforwomen.com.

Gila Films (www.gilafilms.com) • Do-it-yourself Low-E window film.

Glad (www.glad.com) • Glad's food storage products are made from polyethylene (plastic #4) and polypropylene (plastic #5), and contain no PVC, BPA, plasticizers, or dioxins. And no dioxins are formed when heated.

GM (www.gm.com) • Sells FFV and emerging hybrid options under the Chevrolet, Saturn, GMC, and Pontiac brand names. Many of their vehicles also have what is called active fuel management, which means the car only uses all of its engine capacity when it needs it.

Goodman (www.goodmanmfg.com) • Air-source heat pumps and high-SEER-rated air-conditioning systems.

Greasecar (www.greasecar.com) • Do-it-yourself fuel conversion kits that allow your diesel vehicle to run on straight vegetable oil; also has an online list of installation specialists.

Green by Nature (www.greenbynaturebeauty.com) • Personal care products that are 100 percent paraben, DEA, and sulfate free.

Greenfeet (www.greenfeet.com) • Online store with eco-friendly household items.

Green Gift Guide (www.greengiftguide.com) • Links to sites that sell green products and gifts.

Green Home (www.greenhome.com) • An online retailer with a variety of earth-conscious household products.

The Green Loop (www.thegreenloop.com) • Sells stylish eco-friendly clothing and accessories.

GreenOfficeStore.com • An online retailer of green office supplies.

Green to Grow (www.greentogrow.com) • Baby bottles free of phthalates and BPA, and silicone nipples.

Green Works (www.greenworkscleaners.com) • Green cleaning products.

Grounds for Change (www.groundsforchange.com) • Sells coffee that is fair-trade certified, shade grown, and certified organic.

Hansa (www.hansaamerica.net) • High-efficiency faucets with an additional water-limiting feature to use while you are waiting for the water to heat up.

Hansen Living (www.hansenliving.com) • Makes eco-friendly, long-lasting kitchens and bathrooms out of wood that comes from responsibly managed forests.

Hemp Traders (www.hemptraders.com) • Contains lots of great information about hemp and sells hemp fabric.

Hertz (www.hertz.com) • Has higher-fuel-efficiency and hybrid rental vehicles available, including Toyota Priuses.

Hewlett-Packard Company (www.hp.com) • Computers and other office equipment with eco-friendly and energy-saving options like Energy Star ratings, mercury-free displays, and power-saving options.

Home Depot (www.homedepot.com) • Has an Eco Options program and sells many eco-friendly home products and appliances.

Honda Motor Company (www.honda.com) • Sells hybrid and fuel-cell technology vehicles.

Hoover (www.hoover.com) • Has HEPA vacuum cleaners.

Hunter (www.hunterfan.com) • High-quality fans.

Hunter Douglas (www.hunterdouglas.com) • Leader in honeycomb shades and many other window coverings; has a designer screening fabric option with no PVC and no emissions, and is recyclable.

Icynene (www.icynene.com) • Energy Star–rated household insulation that can also be used to easily fill walls in older homes without taking down existing structures or walls.

IKEA (www.ikea.com) • Environmentally conscious vendor of home furnishing products.

Indus-Tool (www.indus-tool.com) • Energy-efficient radiant portable heaters.

Java-Log (www.java-log.com) • Fire logs made from recycled spent coffee grounds and all-natural vegetable wax—100 percent renewable resources—that produce 70–80 percent less emissions than wood.

JELD-WEN (www.jeld-wen.com) • Sells Energy Star–rated, high-quality doors and windows that are energy efficient.

Kenmore (www.kenmore.com) • Home appliances with water-efficiency features and Energy Star ratings.

Kichler Lighting (www.kichler.com) • Energy Star–rated lighting fixtures.

Kimpton Hotels (www.kimptonhotels.com) • Excellent dedication to eco-friendly hotel practices.

Kohler (www.kohler.com) • High-efficiency toilets (including dual flush) and low-flow faucet fixtures.

Kushies (www.kushies.com) • Has fitted cloth diapers and both flushable and washable liners.

Le Creuset (www.lecreuset.com) • Makers of cast-iron cookware.

Lenovo (www.lenovo.com) • Energy Star–rated computer products with energy-efficient and eco-friendly features like lower power consumption, mercury-free LED displays, and are made to be recycled at the end of the product's life.

Lenzing Fibers (www.lenzing.com) • Producers of Tencel fabric—has more information about this fabric in the textile portion of its Web site.

Leviton (www.leviton.com) • Full range of lighting switches, including dimmers and motion sensor switches.

Lexus (www.lexus.com) • Several hybrid vehicle choices including a stylish SUV; Lexus is a division of Toyota.

LG Electronics (www.lge.com) • Has eco-designed appliances and electronics that are focused on efficiency, energy reduction, less hazardous materials in manufacturing, and more recyclability.

Lighting Science Group (www.lsgc.com) • Sells screw-in LED lightbulbs and other quality LED lighting products.

Litebook (www.litebook.com) • Excellent portable light box therapy machines.

Lodge (www.lodgemfg.com) • Makers of cast-iron cookware.

Loomstate Organic (www.loomstate.org) • Organic cotton jeans.

Lowes (www.lowes.com) • Sells Energy Star–rated products.

Lumiram (www.lumiram.com) • Daylight and full-spectrum lighting, including CFLs.

Lutron (www.lutron.com) • High-quality dimmers.

Mansfield Plumbing Products (www.mansfieldplumbing.com) • High-efficiency toilets with the WaterSense label, including dual flush.

Marin (www.marinbikes.com) • High-quality bikes for every kind of rider.

Marriott (www.marriott.com) • International hotel chain has eco-friendly initiatives and goals in energy and water conservation, waste reduction and recycling, and supports community efforts to protect the planet and its habitats.

Maytag (www.maytag.com) • High-efficiency and Energy Star–rated household laundry and kitchen appliances. Maytag is a Whirlpool company.

Mazda (www.mazdausa.com) • Sells the Tribute hybrid SUV.

Merida Meridian (www.meridameridian.com) • Natural fiber woven floor coverings, which include the use of sisal, seagrass, jute, paper, and wool.

Method (www.methodhome.com) • Green cleaning and household products that are widely available and also fully disclose ingredients.

Milliken Carpet (www.millikencarpet.com) • Has green choices for flooring and wall coverings. The company has a recycling program for its customers' carpet tile, saving it from being dumped into landfills.

Minka Group (www.minka.com) • Energy Star–rated lighting fixtures and ceiling fans.

Moen (www.moen.com) • Low-flow, WaterSense-labeled faucets and water-saving showerheads.

Mythic (www.mythicpaint.com) • Sells paint that is noncarcinogenic, with zero VOCs and zero toxins.

NativeEnergy (www.nativeenergy.com) • Multiverified carbon offset program that focuses on building and supporting new, clean, and renewable sources of energy.

NaturaLawn (www.nl-amer.com) • Organic-based lawn care service with franchises throughout the United States.

naturalLee (www.naturallee.com) • Fascinating and fashionable sustainable furniture.

NatureMill (www.naturemill.com) • Compact bugfree composting machine.

NEC Display (www.necdisplay.com) • Energy Star display screens and monitors with a recycling program.

Nestle Waters (www.nestle-watersna.com) • This company has an Eco-Shape bottled water line under several brand names, which uses 30 percent less oil-based plastic than conventional water bottles.

Nissan (www.nissanusa.com) • Sells the Altima hybrid.

NurturePure (www.nurturepure.com) • Sells toxin-free glass baby bottles, and silicone, chemical-free nipples.

Office Depot (www.officedepot.com) • Sells eco-friendly office supplies.

Olympic (www.olympic.com) • Has a line of premium interior paints with zero VOCs and the Green Seal of approval.

Organic Bouquet (www.organicbouquet.com) • Organic flowers and gifts.

Organic to Go (www.organictogo.com) • USDA-certified organic food caterer.

Organic Valley Farms (www.organicvalley.coop) • A nationally distributed farmer-owned co-op of organically produced dairy and other farm products.

Origins (www.originsorganics.com) • USDA Organic certified line of skin, body, and hair care products.

Ott-Lite (www.ott-lite.com) • Daylight lighting lamps, especially good for tasks like reading, sewing, and art.

Panasonic (www.panasonic.com) • Focus on many environmental initiatives, including Energy Star certification, refurbishment of PC notebooks, and electronics recycling.

Patagonia (www.patagonia.com) • Sells a number of durable organic and alternative fabric clothes, as well as clothes made from recycled polyester, and has a Common Threads Recycling Program.

Pelican (www.pelican.com) • Sells virtually indestructible reusable plastic cases that can be used to pack and ship back and forth nearly indefinitely, cutting down on Styrofoam and cardboard use.

People Powered Machines (www.peoplepoweredmachines.com) • Sells manual push mowers and electric mowers.

Phifer (www.phifer.com) • Do-it-yourself solar exterior screens and interior solar shading products.

Philips (www.usa.philips.com) • Electronics, lighting, and smaller appliances and personal care household products.

Physicians Formula (www.organicwearmakeup.com) • Sells Organic Wear line of makeup.

Pine Mountain Logs (www.pinemountainbrands.com) • Clean-burning fire logs.

Pioneer (www.pioneerelectronics.com) • Energy Star-certified electronic products with energy-save mode. Also dedicated to reducing VOCs in its manufacturing and pushing the development of plant-based plastics.

Pizza Fusion (www.pizzafusion.com) • Has a whole host of environmental initiatives, from the sustainability of the food the establishment serves to how it is delivered.

Planet (www.planetinc.com) • Certified biodegradable cleaners and detergents.

Plantoys (www.plantoys.com) • Environmentally friendly toys.

Price Pfister (www.pricepfister.com) • Beautiful WaterSense-labeled low-flow faucets and aerators that can be installed by consumers themselves.

Primo (www.primowater.com) • Bottled water that is in plastic bottles made from plants instead of oil. The bottles can be industrially composted. You can ask your local recycling center if they do industrial composting or you can find a list of industrial composting centers at Primo's Web site, in the Frequently Asked Questions section.

PUR (www.purwaterfilter.com) • Pitcher and faucet-mount at-home water filtration.

PureAyre (www.pureayre.com) • Nontoxic air freshener made from plant-derived enzymes, purified water, and essential oils.

Pure-O-Flow (www.pureoflow.com) • Reverse osmosis system that purifies the water including removing hardness salts so that you get softer water without the chemicals.

Radio Shack (www.radioshack.com) • Sells a variety of rechargeable batteries and chargers.

Rainbird (www.rainbird.com) • Company that has irrigation products, such as timers, sprinklers, valves, and drip systems.

Rentacrate (www.rentacrate.com) • Rentable reusable crates for your moving needs.

Reusable Bags (www.reusablebags.com) • Sells reusable shopping bags, reusable aluminum and stainless steel water bottles, and reusable lunch kits.

Rheem (www.rheemtankless.com) • Tankless water heaters with low emissions features. Also makes solar water heaters: http://waterheating.rheem.com.

Samsung (www.samsung.com) • Extensive green management initiatives to reduce packaging, add power-saving features, and introduce a reusable notebook PC.

Sandals and Beaches Resorts (www.sandals.com) • This resort chain has a written environmental statement, third-party endorsement, and has won awards for its commitment to eco-friendly initiatives.

Saran (www.saranbrands.com) • Plastic food wrap that is free of PVC and BPA, and is also dioxin free so that it can be heated safely in the microwave.

Schwinn (www.schwinnbike.com) • Carries a full line of bicycles including an electric version that can assist the rider for up to sixty miles; the Collegiate Coasting bike is great for moms who have not been on a bike in a while.

Sea Gull Lighting (www.seagulllighting.com) • Ceiling fans with the Energy Star rating.

Seventh Generation (www.seventhgeneration.com) • Excellent line of green-cleaning products, including dish-washing and laundry detergents. Also has chlorine-free disposable diapers, paper towels, and trash bags.

Sherwin-Williams (www.sherwin-williams.com) • Has a Duration Home line of paints with lower VOCs and a Harmony paint line with less solvents and zero VOCs.

SIGG (www.mysigg.com) • Sells high-quality, non-leaching aluminum bottles and containers that are also fasionable.

Simple Green (www.simplegreen.com) • Many useful and widely available green-oriented cleaning products; the company has a link to MSDSs for each product—excellent full disclosure.

Solar Gard (www.solargard.com) • Window films with Low-E and heat control.

SolarWorld (www.solarworld-usa.com) • High-quality solar power modules/systems backed by a twenty-five-year warranty. The company includes recycling efforts in both production of the modules and the product's end of life.

Solatube (www.solatube.com) • Excellent new-generation tubular skylights with an Energy Star rating.

Sony Electronics (www.sony.com) • Dedicated to environmentally friendly new electronics such as eco-friendly notebook computers and low-power-use organic OLED televisions. The company also has extensive electronic recycling efforts underway—more at www.sony.com/recycle.

Springs Window Fashions (Bali, Graber, and Nanik brands) (www.springs windowfashions.com) • Solar shades that block up to 95 percent of heat, have UV block, and low-VOC emissions from the fabric.

Stalk Market (www.stalkmarket.com) • Biodegradable and 100 percent compostable disposable plates, bowls, serving trays, sandwich boxes, cups, and flatware.

Staples (www.staples.com) and (www.staples.com/ecoeasy) • Has many eco-friendly office supplies including thousands of products which incorporate recycled content.

Starch Tech (www.starchtech.com) • 100 percent biodegradable peanut packing material made from corn and potatoes with no petroleum.

St. Gabriel Laboratories (www.milkyspore.com) • Offers a natural weed control made from corn gluten meal and other eco-friendly lawn and garden products.

Stihl (www.stihlusa.com) • Sells backpack and electric blowers, trimmers, and chain saws that have lower emissions engines; also sells nonpetroleum-based oils and lubricants that biodegrade in twenty-one days.

Storopack (www.storopackinc.com) • Variety of environmentally friendly packing materials available with no petroleum plastics in the materials.

Stout (www.bettymills.com) • Eco-friendly trash bag options.

Sylvania (www.sylvania.com) • Full range of energy-efficient lighting including daylight-labeled lighting.

TAM Skylights (www.tamskylights.com) • Energy Star–rated skylights, also available with Low-E and the ability to open up (to improve ventilation).

Target (www.target.com) • This retailer sells a number of reusable shopping bags and totes.

Technical Consumer Products (www.tcpi.com) • Makes a nice warm white CFL lamp that produces light very close to the look of incandescent.

Therma-Tru Doors (www.thermatru.com) • Beautiful Energy Star–rated high-quality doors, including fiberglass; uses a variety of recycled products in its doors, including recycled wood chips, diapers, and plastic bottles.

Thermos (www.thermos.com) • Sells BPA-free, nontoxic beverage bottles made of stainless steel.

Thomas Lighting (www.thomaslighting.com) • Energy Star–rated lighting fixtures.

Toro (www.toro.com) • You can find high-quality irrigation timers, sprinklers, valves, and drip systems from this company.

Toshiba (www.toshiba.com) • Is showing considerable commitment to the environment and public health by phasing PVC and BFR out of *all* of its products and offers to take back and recycle its computers and televisions.

TOTO USA (www.totousa.com) • WaterSense-labeled high-efficiency toilets and faucets, including sensor faucets and dual-flush toilets.

Toyota (www.toyota.com) • Manufacturer of high-quality hybrid vehicles.

Trader Joe's (www.traderjoes.com) • Sells fair-trade coffees, with shade-grown certified-organic varieties, as well as many organic and responsible food choices.

Trane (www.trane.com) • Whole-house air cleaners and ventilation systems, air-source heat pumps, and air conditioners.

Treecycle (www.treecycle.com) • Online catalog of many green office supplies, including recycled papers and biodegradable food service products.

Trex (www.trex.com) • Makes decking, railing, fencing, and trim with reclaimed or recycled safe plastic and wood fibers.

True Flow (www.trueflow.com) • Foam air filters for your car that are reusable.

Tushies (www.tushies.com) • Toxic- and chemical-free diapers.

UPS (www.sustainability.ups.com) • Besides having a ground-shipping service, the shipping company is serious about addressing environmental issues—including operating the greenest vehicle fleet in the shipping industry, using less trucks (equaling less pollution) to deliver, and reusable next day air envelopes which are bleach free and made from 100 percent recycled fiber.

Verilux (www.verilux.com) • Daylight and full-spectrum lighting, including CFLs.

The Vistawall Group (www.vistawall.com) • Has beautiful skylights that not only would save money on energy by lighting your business with the sun but also add beauty to your building.

Wal-Mart (www.walmart.com) • Has a mandatory company policy of increasing its partnerships with local farmers. During the summer months, its grocery stores must purchase one-fifth of its produce from within each store's state.

WaterPik (www.waterpik.com) • Low-flow showerheads.

WeatherTRAK (www.weathertrak.com) • The company provides a weather-tracking irrigation service.

Whirlpool (www.whirlpool.com) • Energy Star–rated appliances for the kitchen, laundry, and whole home.

White Apricot (www.whiteapricot.com) • Online newsletter and portal to fashion and beauty products that are ecologically and socially conscious.

WhiteWing Steamer (www.allergybuyersclubshopping.com) • A steamer for cleaning that has a mop and other attachments to clean nearly all surfaces in your home.

Whole Foods (www.wholefoodsmarket.com) • Large variety of organic products and more eco-friendly coffees.

Xbox (www.xbox.com) • Game console with a sleep mode to conserve energy during long downloads (which can take several hours); and a timer that can be set to restrict the amount of time spent playing games.

Zebra (www.zebra-eco.com) • Has a line of pencils, pens, and highlighters that are made
from 70 percent postconsumer waste materials, like used car headlights, CDs, cell
phones, and plastic bags.

Zipcar (www.zipcar.com) • Car sharing service in major U.S. cities.

Ziploc (www.ziploc.com) • Free of PVC, BPA, and dioxins, this company's plastic food bags
and containers are also formulated not to contain harmful phthalates. The containers are
a plastic #5. The nonsteam and nonslider closure bags are a plastic #4. Other bags with
the slider closure and steaming capability are a mix of plastics numbers 1, 4, and 5—and
therefore would be considered a plastic #7 because of this mix. Plastic #7 is not toxic,
but is considered more difficult to recycle.

OCEAN-FRIENDLY RESOURCES

Got Mercury? (www.gotmercury.org) • Has a mercury calculator online to help you
determine how to make healthier seafood choices.

The Ocean Project (www.theoceanproject.org) • Coordinates a partner network of
aquariums, zoos, and museums, which all believe in and practice ocean conservation.
This Web site also offers ocean-friendly tips.

Seafood Watch (www.seafoodwatch.org) • An indispensable organization to help discern
what is sustainable seafood.

RECYCLING AND WASTE REDUCTION

41 Pounds (www.41pounds.org) • Helps you rid your mailbox of junk mail.

The Center for a New American Dream (www.newdream.org) • Links to reduce junk mail.

Collective Good (www.collectivegood.com) • Recycles mobile phones.

Direct Marketing Association (www.dmaconsumers.org) • Ways to remove yourself from
marketing lists that lead to junk mail.

Earth Easy (www.eartheasy.com) • Online guide for composting.

Ecocycle (www.ecocycle.org) • Nonprofit recycler with many resources and ideas on zero
waste and recycling.

The Freecycle Network (www.freecycle.org) • A grassroots, nonprofit portal that helps
you tap into people who are giving and getting stuff for free.

Gary Liss & Associates (www.garyliss.com) • Unique consulting services for communities
and businesses to help them draft and implement zero-waste plans and resource
recovery.

The Grassroots Recycling Network (www.grrn.org) • Terrific resource for the zero-waste
movement.

Green Dimes (www.greendimes.com) • Service that helps you reduce your junk mail.

HowToCompost (http://howtocompost.org) • Lots of great information about
composting.

Jaco Environmental (www.jacoinc.net) • Curbside appliance recycling pickup.

Recellular (www.recellular.com) • Recycles cell phones, batteries, PDAs, and chargers.

Rechargeable Battery Recycling Corporation (www.call2recycle.org) • Recycles
rechargeable batteries and cell phones.

Reuse Development Organization (REDO) (www.redo.org) • Nonprofit that helps
coordinate surplus building materials for reuse by other organizations.

Share the Technology (www.sharetechnology.org) • Portal to help you find places locally
and nationally where you can donate or recycle your computer equipment.

Staples (www.staples.com) • Accepts used electronics for recycling for a nominal fee,
gives store credit for bringing in used ink cartridges, and offers free collection of cellular

phones, PDAs, pagers, digital cameras, and chargers in conjunction with nonprofit organization efforts.

Virgin Mobile (www.virginmobileusarecycle.com) • Offers a cell phone recycling program.

The Zero Waste International Alliance (www.zwia.org) • A nonprofit organization dedicated to educating, assisting, and being a resource for zero-waste goals of communities and organizations.

SCHOOLS

Airwatch Northwest (www.airwatchnorthwest.org) • Offers an online anti-idling tool kit for reducing emissions at your child's school.

Alliance to Save Energy (www.ase.org) • This nonprofit coalition has a fabulous green schools program to help your school save energy through the efforts of students, faculty, and staff. The program centers around energy efficiency and conservation and includes lesson plans for teachers.

American Society of Heating, Refrigerating, and Air-Conditioning Engineers (ASHRAE) (www.ashrae.org/freeaedg) • This organization has published an energy-saving guide titled *Advanced Energy Design Guide for K–12 School Buildings* that speaks to school engineers but can be a useful resource for you to bring to the attention of your child's school. This guide also addresses the use of daylight lighting.

Blue Bird Corporation (www.blue-bird.com) • Sells propane- and natural gas–powered school buses.

Collaborative for High Performance Schools (www.chps.net) • Oversees a green building rating program for schools K–12.

Community Food Security Coalition (CFSC) (www.foodsecurity.org) • Has information and organizational tools for you to start a farm-to-school program.

EarthTeam (www.earthteam.net) • A network of business and education leaders, which was formed to help San Francisco Bay Area schools and youth go green. There are a lot of ideas about how to green your school and community, and how to get youth to participate.

Farm to School (www.farmtoschool.org) • This is a great resource for you if you want to get a farm-to-school program started in your child's school or school district.

The Fruit Tree Planting Foundation (www.ftpf.org) • A nonprofit charity dedicated to planting fruit trees in low-income schools.

Funding Factory (www.fundingfactory.com) • A printer cartridge and cell phone recycling program to be used as a fundraiser.

The Green Flag Program (www.greenflagschools.org) • A program to help change environmental behaviors at your child's school.

Greenraising (www.greenraising.com) • An alternative school fundraising resource that advocates products that consume less, preserve natural resources, and help others.

IC Bus (www.icbus.com) • Sells hybrid school buses.

The IPM Institute of North America (www.ipminstitute.org/school.htm) • A nonprofit organization dedicated to reducing pesticides and, instead, practicing integrated pest management (IPM). IPM reduces or eliminates conventional pesticides and instead concentrates efforts on prevention and more ecologically friendly ways of managing pests. IPM practices can make your child's school environment safer.

Laptop Lunches (www.laptoplunches.com) • Sells practical lunch containers and offers guides on how to make your child's school lunch healthier.

Lowe's (www.lowes.com) • Has an outdoor classroom grant program to help you find funds for a school garden.

National Garden Association (www.kidsgardening.org) • This kid-oriented site of the NGA has lots of help for parents, volunteers, and teachers in starting up and maintaining a school garden.

National Sustainable Agriculture Information Service (www.attra.ncat.org) • Offers a great online guide titled *Bringing Local Food to Local Institutions: A Resource Guide for Farm-to-Schools and Farm-to-Institutions Programs*.

Organic Consumers Association (www.organicconsumers.org/afc) • Has an environmental health campaign that aims to rid schools of pesticides, transition school lunches toward healthier and more organic options, and teach children about sustainable agriculture.

Oregon Green Schools (www.oregongreenschools.org) • A nonprofit organization that helps Oregon schools go green. If you don't live in Oregon, use this to generate ideas for your area.

Reusable Planet (www.reusableplanetonline.com) • Provides refilled printing cartridges for school fundraising efforts.

Roots and Shoots (www.rootsandshoots.org) • Environmentally focused youth program started by the legendary animal activist Jane Goodall.

Setting Up and Running a School Garden (www.fao.org) • This helpful online guide is published by the Food and Agricultural Organization of the United Nations—type in the title of the guide in the site's search bar to find the link.

Tomra (www.tomra.com) • Provides redemption programs for school fundraising.

Walk to School (www.walktoschool.org) • This fabulous site provides information and motivation on walking or riding a bike to school.

WAL-MART Kids Recycling Challenge (www.kidsrecyclingchallenge.com) • A program that teaches elementary school students about the importance of recycling while earning money for their schools.

Waste-Free Lunches (www.wastefreelunches.org) • Info to help you create a waste-free school lunch for your child.

YoNaturals (www.yonaturals.com) • Provider of vending machines with healthier food options, including organic products.

TAKE-ACTION ORGANIZATIONS

Alaska Wilderness League (www.alaskawild.org) • Helps protect Alaska's public lands.

Algalita Marine Research Foundation (www.algalita.org) • Does marine research, education, and restoration.

American Bird Conservancy (www.abcbirds.org) • Conserves native wild birds and their habitats throughout the Americas.

American Forests (www.americanforests.org) • Focuses on planting trees for environmental restoration.

American Rivers (www.americanrivers.org) • Offers river cleanups.

Arbor Day Foundation (www.arborday.org) • Promotes planting and caring for trees.

Beyond Pesticides (www.beyondpesticides.org) • Promotes a pesticide-free world.

Center for Health, Environment & Justice (www.chej.org) • Has helpful campaigns and information that help protect you and your family from exposure to dangerous environmental chemicals.

Clean Ocean Action (www.cleanoceanaction.org) • Helps protect waterways, oceans, and beaches.

Clean Water Action (www.cleanwateraction.org) • Provides information about legislation that can affect your water supply and the environment.

Clean Water Fund (www.cleanwaterfund.org) • Promotes cleaner and safer water, cleaner air, and protection from toxic pollution in our homes, neighborhoods, and workplaces.

Conservation International (www.conservation.org) • Concerned with environmental issues including biodiversity and protecting endangered regions and waters.

Defenders of Wildlife (www.defenders.org) • Promotes wildlife conservation.

Earth Day Network (www.earthday.net) • The main Web site for Earth Day and year-round environmental awareness programs.

Earth Hour (www.earthhour.org) • A campaign by the World Wildlife Fund (www.wwf.org) that encourages residents and businesses to turn off their lights when not in use. Every year there is a promotional earth hour when everyone across the globe is encouraged to turn off their lights to send a message about climate awareness.

Earthjustice (www.earthjustice.org) • Helps solve environmental actions pro bono.

Earth Share (www.earthshare.org) • Encourages businesses to support environmental initiatives.

Environmental Defense (www.edf.org) • Partners with businesses and communities to help the environment.

Environmental Media Association (www.ema-online.org) • Mobilizes the entertainment industry in educating people about environmental issues.

Fauna & Flora International (www.fauna-flora.org)   Works to preserve biodiversity.

ForestEthics (www.forestethics.org) • Protects endangered forests and has a number of tools and resources online to help you implement a forest-friendly purchasing policy.

Global Green USA (www.globalgreen.org) • Founded by Mikhail S. Gorbachev, it offers climate change and clean drinking water initiatives.

Go Green Initiative (www.gogreeninitiative.org) • Offers guidelines on helping schools become more green.

Greenpeace (www.greenpeace.org) • Has initiatives and education about eliminating toxic chemicals in our environment.

Healing Our Waters—Great Lakes Coalition (www.healthylakes.org) • Helps raise awareness to clean up the Great Lakes.

Heal the Bay (www.healthebay.org) • Works to keep California's beaches clean.

The Humane Society of the United States (www.hsus.org) • Promotes healthy habitats and sustainable initiatives.

International Dark-Sky Association (www.darksky.org) • Preserves and protects the nighttime environment.

Keep America Beautiful (www.kab.org) • Connects you with volunteer opportunities to help improve your community's environment.

League of American Bicyclists (www.bikeleague.org) • Promotes bicycling for fun, fitness, transportation, and work.

League of Conservation Voters (www.lcv.org) • A policy organization as well as a resource to find your representatives and senators and learn how they score on voting for or against environmental issues.

Mangrove Action Project (www.mangroveactionproject.org) • Encourages protection and better management of coastal environments and tackles abuses in the shrimp industry.

National Audubon Society (www.audubon.org) • Conserves and restores natural eco-systems, with a special focus on birds.

National Parks Conservation Association (www.npca.org) • An advocate group for U.S. national parks.

National Wildlife Federation (www.nwf.org) • Inspires Americans to protect wildlife for our children's future. Has a certified wildlife habitat program for consumers. And the organization has a fabulous green hour program that encourages kids to get outdoor time for health and happiness—see www.greenhour.org.

Natural Resources Defense Council (www.nrdc.org) • Advocates safeguarding the environment.

The Nature Conservancy (www.nature.org) • Organization works around the world to protect ecologically important lands and waters.

Non-GMO Project (www.nongmoproject.org) • Information about genetically modified foods and an emerging non-GMO verification standard.

Office of the Federal Environmental Executive (www.ofee.gov) • A White House task force on waste prevention and recycling.

Organic Consumers Association (www.organicconsumers.org) • Offers useful information about organic products.

Organic Trade Association (www.ota.com) • Protects and promotes organic trade for farmers and the public.

Parent-Teacher Association (www.pta.org) • National parent-teacher advocacy group.

Pedestrian and Bicycle Information Center (www.pedbikeinfo.org) • Promotes safe walking and bicycling.

Points of Light and Hands On Network (www.handsonnetwork.org) • Connects volunteers across the United States.

Pollution Prevention Center (http://departments.oxy.edu/uepi/ppc/consumer.htm) • A division of the Urban and Environmental Policy Institute of Occidental College in Los Angeles; actively promoting public awareness of better choices when it comes to dry cleaning.

Sierra Club (www.sierraclub.org) • Advocates protecting the environment locally and globally.

Silicon Valley Toxics Coalition (www.etoxics.org) • Promotes safety with high-tech products.

Slow Food (www.slowfoodusa.org) • Promotes an environmentally sustainable food system.

Surfrider Foundation (www.surfrider.org) • Helps protect our oceans and beaches.

Sustainable Furniture Council (www.sustainablefurniturecouncil.org) • Promotes sustainable furniture options.

Sustainable Sites Initiative (www.sustainablesites.org) • Promotes sustainable and eco-friendly landscapes.

Union of Concerned Scientists (www.ucsusa.org) • Scientists and citizens focusing on ways science can help the planet.

Urban Land Institute (www.uli.org) • Promotes responsible use of land.

Volunteer Match (www.volunteermatch.org) • Matches up volunteers with nonprofits and businesses with businesses' civic activities.

Washington Toxics Coalition (www.watoxics.org) • Advocates for safer products, including lead-free toys.

Waterkeeper Alliance (www.waterkeeper.org) • Promotes clean water.

Wildcoast (www.wildcoast.net) • Protects coastal ecosystems and their wildlife.

Women's Voices for the Earth (www.womenandenvironment.org) • This women's environmental organization has a Host a Green Cleaning Party program where you and your friends get together to make your own nontoxic cleaning products.

World Resources Institute (www.wri.org) • An environmental think tank that finds practical ways to protect the earth and improve people's lives.

World Wildlife Fund (www.wwf.org) • The largest conservation organization in the world.

TOXIC CHEMICAL INFORMATION

Pollution in People (www.pollutioninpeople.org) • Information on toxic chemicals and safer alternatives.

Tox Town (www.toxtown.nlm.nih.gov) • An interactive Web site of the U.S. National Library of Medicine that helps you identify environmental health concerns in your area.

TRANSPORTATION

CarSharing.net (www.carsharing.net) • Nonprofit organization that connects you with car-sharing companies in your area.

E85 Prices (www.e85prices.com) • Shows the difference on a U.S. map in current prices between E85 and gasoline fuels.

Edmunds.com (www.edmunds.com) • Prints a yearly online hybrid buying guide.

FuelEconomy.gov (www.fueleconomy.gov) • A great tool for comparing vehicles and how they use fuel—efficiently or not.

Green Vehicle Guide (www.epa.gov/greenvehicle) • An online guide put out by the EPA. You can look up vehicles and make comparisons.

TRAVEL AND RECREATION

Adventure Cycling Association (www.adventurecycling.org) • Cycling info.

American Recreation Coalition (www.funoutdoors.com) • Nonprofit organization that promotes outdoor recreational opportunities.

BicyclingInfo.org (www.bicyclinginfo.org) • Motivational and informational site on biking.

Bikestation (www.bikestation.org) • A not-for-profit organization that offers secure bicycle parking and related services.

Blue Flag (www.blueflag.org) • An organization certifying eco-friendly beaches and marinas in Europe, South Africa, Morocco, New Zealand, Canada, and the Caribbean.

California Agritourism Database (www.calagtour.org) • State-by-state database of agriculture-oriented tourism sites.

Charity Guide (www.charityguide.org) • This nonprofit has a link to a number of environmental volunteer vacation ideas.

Climate Friendly (www.climatefriendly.com) • Carbon offset program with the Gold Standard third-party verification and a philosophy of reduce, renew, and neutralize.

Earthwatch Institute (www.earthwatch.org) • Volunteer opportunities that focus on collecting field data for scientific environmental research.

Environmentally Friendly Hotels (www.environmentallyfriendlyhotels.com) • Online resource for green hotels.

Florida Department of Environmental Protection (www.dep.state.fl.us) • Has several eco-friendly programs to promote the health of the environment and recognize sustainable tourism, including its green lodging program.

Geocaching.com (www.geocaching.com) • Global GPS cache hunt site.

Gold Standard (www.cdmgoldstandard.org) • A certification standard for the carbon offsetting industry.

Green Hotels Association (www.greenhotels.com) • Online resource for green hotels.

Green Vacation Hub (www.greenvacationhub.com) • Online referral service for green travel and hospitality.

Habitat for Humanity (www.habitat.org) • Volunteer vacation opportunities.

Leave No Trace (www.lnt.org) • A fabulous nonprofit organization dedicated to outdoor responsibility.

Maine Farm Vacation Association (www.mainefarmvacation.com) • Bed-and-breakfasts in a rural setting.

My Climate (www.my-climate.com) • Carbon offset program that helps travelers and travel-related companies protect the environment.

Pennsylvania Farm Vacation Association (www.pafarmstay.com) • Member farms with vacation programs.

Planeta.com (www.planeta.com) • Articles about and resource links for eco-tourism.

Rails-to-Trails Conservancy (www.railtrails.org) • Nonprofit organization that turns unused rail corridors into biking and walking trails.

Trip Advisor (www.tripadvisor.com) • Advice site with traveler reviews of travel destinations, accommodations, and restaurants.

WalkingInfo.org (www.walkinginfo.org) • Excellent site to motivate you to walk.

Wilderness Volunteers (www.wildernessvolunteers.org) • Volunteer vacations where you restore public lands.

WATER CONSERVATION

H₂OUSE (www.h2ouse.org) • A terrific water conservation site for consumers by the California Urban Water Conservation Council that helps you learn how to be water wise.

WaterSense (www.epa.gov/watersense) • A new EPA labeling and certification program for water-efficient products.

WORK

Earth Share (www.earthshare.org) • An organization that can help your business set up programs to support environmental initiatives.

Greenbusiness.net (www.greenbusiness.net) • This is a helpful forum for networking and finding out how other businesses are going green.

Responsible Purchasing Network (www.responsiblepurchasing.org) • Offers many resources for companies to learn more about environmentally friendly purchasing.

MEDIA, MAGAZINES, BOOKS, AND FILMS

The 11th Hour: An important documentary by Leonardo DiCaprio that highlights environmental issues and offers solutions.

Clean House Clean Planet by Karen Logan (Pocket—1997). A fabulous book, especially for moms on a budget, on green cleaning. Has lots of cleaner recipes and how-to's.

Condé Nast Traveler (www.concierge.com) • A travel magazine that covers sustainable eco-tourism destinations and services.

Earth: The Sequel by Fred Krupp and Miriam Horn (W.W. Norton & Company—2008). Covers environmental innovations and ideas and how best to implement them.

Environmental Film Festival (www.dcenvironmentalfilmfest.org) • This annual festival in Washington, D.C., shows shorts and feature films that inspire eco-friendly change.

Erin Brockovich: An inspiring film, starring Julia Roberts, about the real-life story of Erin Brockovich who battled the Pacific Gas and Electric Company's industrial poisoning of a town's water supply.

The Great Kapok Tree: A Tale of the Amazon Rain Forest by Lynne Cherry (Voyager Books—2000). A beautiful picture book about saving the rain forests.

The Green Guide (www.thegreenguide.com) • This quarterly magazine produced by National Geographic is an extension of its online resource, which offers tons of great green-living tips.

Grist (www.grist.org) • Provides both environmental news and humor.

Happy Feet: A family film for all ages that touches on environmental themes.

How Groundhog's Garden Grew by Lynne Cherry (Blue Sky Press—2003). A lovely little children's book that encourages kids to garden.

How to Grow Fresh Air by Dr. B. C. Wolverton (Penguin—1997). Excellent reference guide on fifty houseplants that can clean your home or office's indoor air.

An Inconvenient Truth: Unequivocally the most important film you should watch about our changing environment. It helps you understand how global warming has happened and what can be done about it. The film's Web site at www.climatecrisis.net has a lot of follow-up information about the science of global warming.

In Defense of Food: An Eater's Manifesto by Michael Pollan (The Penguin Press HC—2008). The author's mantra here is "Eat food. Not too much. Mostly plants."

Last Child in the Woods: Saving Our Children from Nature-Deficit Disorder by Richard Louv (Algonquin Books—2005). A book that inspires you to get your children outdoors.

The Lorax by Dr. Seuss (Random House Books for Young Readers—1971). Classic children's book about caring for our planet. Includes the memorable quote, "Unless someone like you cares a whole awful lot, nothing is going to get better. It's not."

Manufactured Landscapes: This thought-provoking documentary captures landscape changes due to industrialization in China. It received the Best Canadian Film award at the 2006 Toronto Film Festival.

Momentum magazine (www.momentumplanet.com) • Online cycling resource.

Mountainfilm Festival (www.mountainfilm.org) • Annual film festival in Telluride, Colorado, that aims to educate and inspire about important issues including the environment.

National Geographic (www.nationalgeographic.com) • Educating and inspiring you to learn about your planet.

Natural Home (www.naturalhomemagazine.com) • Magazine focused on earth-friendly living.

Permission to Play by Jill Murphy Long (Sourcebooks—2003). An eye-opening book to help inspire you and give you ideas on how to reawaken your love of play.

Plenty (www.plentymag.com) • Magazine that has lots of well-thought-out eco information, articles, and tips for the average consumer.

The Rodale Book of Composting: Easy Methods for Every Gardener by Grace Gershuny and Deborah L. Martin (Rodale—1992). Everything you could ever want to know about composting.

The Sea, the Storm, and the Mangrove Tangle by Lynne Cherry (Farrar, Straus and Giroux—2004). Beautiful picture book that traces the life of a mangrove.

Six Arguments for a Greener Diet (Center for Science in the Public Interest—2006). A book by scientists who discuss how "eating more plant foods and fewer fatty animal products can lead to extra years of healthy living."

When Your Body Gets the Blues by Dr. Marie-Annette Brown (Rodale Books—2002). Excellent resource for understanding how light affects your health and natural ways of how to avoid seasonal affective disorder (SAD).

The World Without Us by Alan Weisman (St. Martin's Press—2007). What might happen to the earth if humans suddenly ceased to exist.

NOTES

INTRODUCTION

Usability Sciences underwritten by DisneyFamily.com. Survey on eco issues. (Conducted online in 2008 at DisneyFamily.com, with participants being more than 8,000 moms and dads.) The margin of error was ±5 percent; 77 percent of respondents were married, most of the respondents were between the ages of twenty-five and fifty-four, and 88 percent of respondents had between one and three children.

"Lifestyle Choices Affect U.S. Impact on the Environment," Population Reference Bureau, October 2006 Symposium, www.prb.org/Articles/2006/LifestyleChoicesAffectUS Impacton the Environment.aspx.

I. EARTH-FRIENDLY ENERGY

Lenny Bernstein et al., "Climate Change 2007: Synthesis Report" presented at an Intergovernmental Panel on Climate Change press conference, Valencia, Spain, November 17, 2007, www.ipcc.ch/pdf/assessment-report/ar4/syr/ar4_syr.pdf. Additional climate change reports and information are available at www.ipcc.ch.

"The Economics of a Solar Water Heater," *A Consumer's Guide to Energy Efficiency and Renewable Energy,* U.S. Department of Energy, September 12, 2005, www.eere.energy .gov/consumer/your_home/water_heating/index.cfm/mytopic=12860.

2. EARTH-WISE WATER AND LIGHTING

Ben Block, "Lighting an Efficient Future, Minus the Mercury," online article for Worldwatch Institute, May 30, 2008, www.worldwatch.org/node/5757.

"National Lighting Bureau Weighs in on Mercury in Compact Fluorescent (CFL) Lighting," online announcement made by the National Lighting Bureau, Silver Spring, MD, April 22, 2008, www.nlb.org/index.cfm?cdid=10516&pid=10237.

4. CLEAN GREEN

"Composting," U.S. Environmental Protection Agency, September 7, 2007, www.epa.gov/ compost/.

"Children at Risk" report, the Clean Air Task Force, Boston, MA, May 2002, www.catf.us/ publications/reports/Children_at_Risk.pdf.

"Are our children too clean?" *Scotsman,* April 29, 2008, Features section.

S. Hartman, "Antibacterials and Disinfectants: Are They Necessary?" Children's Health Environmental Coalition, www.checnet.org/healthehouse/education/articles-detail.asp? Main_ID=121.

Allison E. Aiello et al., "Antibacterial Cleaning Products and Drug Resistance," Emerging Infectious Diseases, October 2005, vol. 11, no. 10, www.cdc.gov/eid.

5. YOUR GREEN GARDEN

"Cultivating a New Generation of Gardeners," the National Gardening Association, http:// assoc.garden.org/press/press.php?q=show&id=2684&pr=pr_kids.

"A Room with a View Helps Rural Children Deal with Life's Stresses," Cornell University press release, April 24, 2003, www.news.cornell.edu/releases/April03/nature.kid.stress.ssl.html.

"Gardening for Butterflies," a brochure by the Humane Society of the United States, Washington, D.C., 2003.

"Backyard Feeding of Wild Birds," a brochure by the Humane Society of the United States, Washington, D.C., 1996.

6. EAT, DRESS, SPEND GREEN

Hilary Oliver, "Walmart goes a little local," *Natural Foods Merchandiser,* July 31, 2008, http://naturalfoodsmerchandiser.com/tabid/66/itemid/3146/Walmart-goes-a-little-local.aspx.

"Food Labeling: Meat and Poultry Labeling Terms," online fact sheet, United States Department of Agriculture's Food Safety and Inspection Service, August, 24, 2006, www.fsis.usda.gov/FactSheets/Meat_&_Poultry_Labeling_Terms/index.asp.

Charlene Bruce, President of the Association of Food and Drug Officials, letter to U.S. Department of Agriculture's Food Safety and Inspection Service, January 9, 2007, www.afdo.org/afdo/position/2007-Papers.cfm.

"'Natural' on the Label Can be Misleading: Turns Out, It Doesn't Mean Very Much," ConsumerAffairs.com, July 1, 2008, www.consumeraffairs.com/news04/2008/07/natural_food.html.

"Chemical Used to Make Non-Stick Coatings Harmful to Health," Environment News Service, Washington, D.C., May 13, 2008, www.ens-newswire.com/ens/may2008/2008-05-13-093.asp.

Glenn Hurowitz, "Clean Hair or Clean Air?" *Los Angeles Times,* Opinion section, May 19, 2008, p. A15.

Henning Steinfeld et al., "Livestock's Long Shadow: Environmental Issues and Options," United Nations Food and Agriculture Organization report, Rome, Italy, November 29, 2006, www.virtualcentre.org/en/library/key_pub/longshad/A0701E00.htm. Also visit Food and Agriculture Organization's main Web site, at www.fao.org.

Brad Knickerbocker, "Humans' Beef with Livestock: A Warmer Planet," *The Christian Science Monitor,* February 20, 2007.

"Report: Seafood Faces Collapse by 2048," Associated Press, November 3, 2006, www.cnn.com.

"Prescription Drugs Found in Drinking Water Across U.S.," Associated Press, March 10, 2008, www.cnn.com/2008/HEALTH/03/10/pharma.water1/index.html.

7. GREEN ON THE GO

Robert Sullivan, "Air Supply," *Vogue,* July 2008, p. 132.

Lisa Stiffler, "Bio-debatable: Food vs. Fuel," *Seattle Post-Intelligencer,* May 3, 2008, http://seattlepi.nwsource.com/local/361634_biodiesel03.html.

Amy Novotney, "Getting Back to the Great Outdoors," *Monitor on Psychology,* March 2008, vol. 39, no. 3, p. 52, www.apa.org/monitor/2008/03/outdoors.html.

Sarah Mahoney, "The Fresh-Air Fix: The Simple Way to Boost Brainpower, Improve Health, and Feel Great? Spend Time Outside," *Prevention,* www.prevention.com.

"About Green Hour," National Wildlife Federation, www.greenhour.org/section/about (accessed online in April 2008).

Anja Kollmuss and Benjamin Bowell, "Voluntary Offsets for Air-Travel Carbon Emissions: Evaluations and Recommendations of Voluntary Offset Companies," Tufts Climate Initiative, Tufts University, Medford, MA, Revision 1.3, April 5, 2007, www.tufts.edu/tie/tci/pdf/TCI_Carbon_Offsets_Paper_April-2-07.pdf.

8. THE GREEN-COLLAR WORKFORCE

Patricia Calkins, "Smarter Ways to Green: How to Make Sustainability Succeed in Your Business," white paper, Xerox Corporation, February 2008.

Rachel Oliver, "All About: Recycling," CNN, February 4, 2008, http://edition.cnn.com/2008/WORLD/asiapcf/02/03/eco.about.recycling/index.html.

"MEW Light Study Release: New Study Finds That Office Light Increases Employee Performance," press release about a newly completed study by Circadian Technologies, Inc., and Matsushita Electric Works, Ltd., May 5, 2004, at www.circadian.com/media/MEW %20Light%20Study%20release.htm.

"Computers Left On at Night Cost U.S. Businesses $1.7 Billion, Says Study," reprinted from GreenerComputing.com at Lifestyles of Health and Sustainability Online, June 22, 2007, www.lohas.com/articles/100422.html.

9. YOUR GREEN COMMUNITY

"Daylight Lighting in Schools: An Investigation into the Relationship Between Daylighting and Human Performance, Condensed Report," Heschong Mahone Group, Fair Oaks, CA, August 20, 1999, www.h-m-g.com/downloads/Daylighting/schoolc.pdf.

"Windows and Classrooms: A Study of Student Performance and the Indoor Environment: Technical Report," Heschong Mahone Group for the California Energy Commission, Fair Oaks, CA, October 2003, www.h-m-g.com/downloads/Daylighting/A-7_Windows_Classrooms_2.4.10.pdf.

Mark Schneider, "Do School Facilities Affect Academic Outcomes?" National Clearinghouse for Educational Facilities, Washington, D.C., November 2002, www.edfacilities.org/pubs/outcomes.pdf.

John McCreery and Timothy Hill, "Illuminating the Classroom Environment," School Planning and Management, February 2005, vol. 44, pp. 34–36, 38, 39.

Robbin M. Rittner-Heir, "Color and Light in Learning," *School Planning and Management,* February 2002, vol. 41, pp. 57–58, 60–61.

Davidson Norris and Linnaea Tillett, "Daylight and Productivity: Is There a Causal Link?" paper presented at the Sixth International Conference on Architectural and Automotive Glass, Tampere, Finland, June 13–16, 1999, www.glassprocessingdays.com/1999/art2_213.htm.

Patricia Plympton et al., "Daylighting in Schools: Improving Student Performance and Health at a Price Schools Can Afford," presented at the American Solar Energy Society Conference, Madison, WI, June 16, 2000, www.deptplanetearth.com/nrel_student_performance.htm.

Daniel McQuillen, "The Art of Daylighting," Environmental Design + Construction, January 16, 2001, www.edcmag.com.

"Energy-Smart Building Choices: How School Administrators and Board Members Are Improving Learning and Saving Money," U.S. Department of Energy, Office of Building Technology, State and Community Programs, Energy Efficiency and Renewable Energy, August 2001, www.nrel.gov/docs/fy01osti/30558.pdf.

Bill Toland, "A 'Green' School Saves on Costs of Energy," *Pittsburgh Post-Gazette,* August 30, 2004, www.post-gazette.com/pg/04243/370074-85.stm.

"Highlighting High Performance: Clearview Elementary School, Hanover, Pennsylvania," U.S. Department of Energy, National Renewable Energy Laboratory, Golden, CO, August 1, 2002, www.nrel.gov/docs/fy02osti/32680.pdf.

Jeffery A. Lackney, "The Relationship Between Environmental Quality of School Facilities and Student Performance," congressional briefing to the U.S. House of Representatives

Committee on Science sponsored by the Environmental Energy Study Institute, Washington, D.C., September 23, 1999, www.edi.msstate.edu/articlesEnergy.php.

Paula J. Vincent, "Modern Public School Facilities: Investing in the Future," testimony provided to the Committee on Education and Labor, U.S. House of Representatives, Washington, D.C., February 13, 2008, http://edlabor.house.gov/testimony/2008-02-13-PaulaVincent.pdf.

"Growing Cooler: Evidence on Urban Development and Climate Change—Overview," report by the Urban Land Institute, September 20, 2007, www.uli.org.

"Building Lean, Green Businesses and Organizations," zero-waste forum at the Burbank City Council Chamber, Burbank, CA, May 2, 2008.